Pocket Guide to
Clinica
Examination
second edition

Owen Epstein MBBCh FRCP
Consultant Physician & Gastroenterologist
Clinical Tutor & Director of Endoscopy Unit
Royal Free Hospital NHS Trust,
London, UK

G David Perkin BA MB FRCP
Consultant Neurologist
Charing Cross Hospital and Hillingdon Hospital, London, UK

David P de Bono MA MD FRCP
British Heart Foundation Professor of Cardiology and Head of the
Department of Medicine and Therapeutics, University of Leicester.
Clinical Sciences Wing, Glenfield Hospital NHS Trust, Leicester, UK

John Cookson MD FRCP
Consultant Physician & Clinical Sub-Dean (University of Leicester)
Department of Respiratory Medicine
Glenfield Hospital NHS Trust, Leicester, UK

With contributions from:

Neil Solomons MBChB FRCS
Consultant Surgeon in Otolaryngology
Head, Neck and Facial Plastic Surgery
Royal Surrey County Hospital NHS Trust,
Guildford, UK

Andrew Robins MB MSc MRCP FRCPCH
Consultant Paediatrician
Whittington Hospital NHS Trust,
London, UK

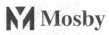 Mosby

London   Philadelphia   St. Louis   Sydney   Tokyo

D0546324

Project Manager:	Jane Tozer
Development Editor:	Gina Almond
Designer:	Paul Phillips
Layout Artist:	Paul Phillips
Cover Design:	Greg Smith
Illustration:	Danny Pyne
Production:	Hamish Adamson
Index:	Anita Reid
Publisher:	Richard Furn

Printed by Printer Trento s.r.l., Trento, Italy

ISBN 0 7234 2577 9

For full details of all Times Mirror International Publishers Limited titles, please write
to Times Mirror International Publishers Limited, Lynton House, 7–12 Tavistock
Square, London WC1H 9LB, England.

A CIP catalogue record for this book is available from the British Library.
Library of Congress Cataloging-in-Publication Data Applied For

Preface

The Pocket Guide to Clinical Examination second edition is a handy reference based on the parent textbook in this series, Clinical Examination second edition. It contains the core information required to conduct a thorough history and examination. Like the parent textbook this pocket guide is illustrated and includes numerous "icon" boxes which both summarise important information and offer a frame-work for rapid revision.

The pocket guide is one of four publications in the Clinical Examination Compendium.The combination of Clinical Examination second edition, CD-ROM Clinical Examination, Case Studies in Clinical Examination second edition and this book, Pocket Guide to Clinical Examination second edition offers the complete collection of learning and teaching material for students of clinical medicine.

Icon Boxes

 Questions to Ask Boxes – key questions to ask the patient to help reach a diagnosis

 Disorder Boxes – summaries of the disorders that can occur within each body system and their possible causes

 Emergency Boxes – implications for history and examination of certain clinical emergencies

 Summary Boxes – key points of clinical relevance

 Risk Factor Boxes – basic information on the risk factors associated with particular diseases

 Examination of Elderly People Boxes – particular difficulties and differences encountered when examining the elderly

Contents

1. Medical Record, Medical History and Interviewing Technique

Before setting out to learn about clinical examination, it is important to know how to write up a full medical record. The initial record will include a detailed history and examination as well as plans for investigation and treatment. Whenever the results of investigations become available, this new information is added to the record and at each follow-up visit, progress and change in management are recorded.

PROBLEM-ORIENTATED MEDICAL RECORD

The accuracy of information gathered from a patient during the course of an illness influences the precision of the diagnosis and treatment.

The problem-orientated medical record (POMR) provides a framework for standardising the structure of follow-up notes; this stresses changes in the patient's symptoms and signs and the evolution of clinical assessment and management plans. The POMR also provides a flow sheet that is designed to record sequential changes in clinical and biochemical measurements.

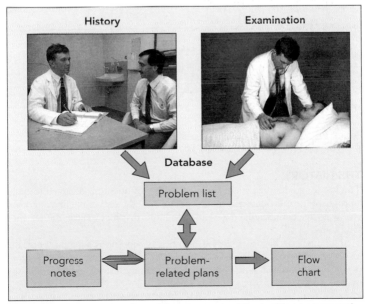

Diagrammatic representation of the structure of the problem-orientated medical record (POMR).

No	active problems	date	inactive problems	date
1	jaundice (Jan '97)	9/1/97		
2	anorexia (Dec '96)	9/1/97		
3	weight loss	9/1/97		
4	recurrent rectal bleeding	9/1/97		
5	smoking (since 1970)	9/1/97		
6	unemployed (Nov '96)	9/1/97		
7	stutter	9/1/97		
8			duodenal ulcer (1966)	9/1/97
9				
10				

Patient's name: Hospital No:

Problem list entered on 9 January 1997.

THE HISTORY

The history guides the patient through a series of questions designed to build a profile of the individual and their problems. By the end of the first interview you will have considered a differential diagnosis that may explain the patient's symptoms.

The medical history involves a series of questions ranging from the presenting complaint to the social history, education, employment history, personal habits, travel, home circumstances, family history and review of the major systems.

THE EXAMINATION

The examination may confirm or refute a diagnosis suspected from the history and by adding this information to the database you will be able to construct a more accurate problem list. The examination is structured to record both positive and negative findings in detail.

THE PROBLEM LIST

The problem list is fundamental to the POMR. The entries provide a record of all the patient's important health-related problems. In addition to providing a summary and index, the problem list also assists in the development of management plans.

Setting up the problem list

Divide the problems into those that are active (or require action) and those that are inactive (problems that have resolved or require no action but may be important at some stage in the patient's present or future management).

Your entries into the problem list may include established diagnoses (e.g. ulcerative colitis), symptoms (e.g. dyspnoea), physical signs (e.g. ejection systolic murmur), laboratory tests (e.g. anaemia), psychological and social history (e.g. depression, unemployment, parental or marital problems) or special risk factors (e.g. smoking, alcohol or narcotic abuse).

The problem list is designed to accommodate change, consequently, it is not necessary to delete an entry once a higher level of diagnosis (or understanding) is reached. The problem list should be under constant review to ensure that the entries are accurate and up to date.

INITIAL PROBLEM-RELATED PLANS

By constructing the problem list you will have clearly defined problems requiring active management (i.e. investigation and treatment), so it should be reasonably easy to develop a plan for each problem by considering four headings:

Diagnostic tests (Dx)
Monitoring tests (Mx)
Treatment (Rx)
Education (Ed)

PROGRESS NOTES

The POMR provides a disciplined and standardised structure to the follow-up note. There are four headings to guide you through the progress note:

Subjective (S)
Objective (O)
Assessment (A)
Plan (P)

FLOW CHARTS

Clinical investigations and measurements are often repeated to monitor the course of acute or chronic illness. A flow sheet is convenient for recording these data in a format which, at a glance, provides a summary of trends and progress. Graphs may be equally revealing.

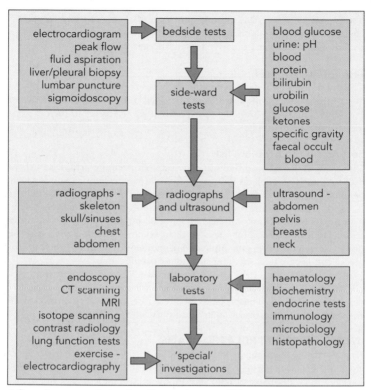

A flow diagram to help plan diagnostic tests. (CT, computerised tomography; MRI, magnetic resonance imaging.)

A flow chart is a convenient method for recording results of tests because it summarises trends and progress.

CONFIDENTIALITY

Clinical notes contain confidential information and it is of vital importance that you protect this confidentiality.

INTERVIEWING TECHNIQUES AND HISTORY-TAKING

Studies indicate that over 80% of diagnoses in general medical clinics are

Date	9.1.97	11.1.97	13.1.97	14.1.97	7.2.97	14.2.97
Tests						
Bilirubin (<17)	233	190	130		28	10
AST (<40)	1140	830	500		52	23
ALT (<45)	1600	650	491		61	31
Albumin (35–45)	41	40	41	d	42	43
Pro-time (s)	14/12	14/12	13/12	i s c h a r g e	13/12	12/12
Haemoglobin (11.5–16.2)	12.1	12.3	12.1		12.2	12.6
Blood urea (3.5–6.5)	3.1	4.2	4.8		6.0	6.2
Blood glucose (3.5–6.5)	5.5	6.8	5.0		5.6	6,0
Hepatitis screen			IgM Hep A +ve			
Cholesterol (3.5–6.8)			8.1			8.4

An example of a flow sheet. (ALT, alanine transaminase, AST, aspartate transaminase.)

based on the interview. It is clear that the way in which the interview is conducted and the type of questions asked determine the amount of diagnostically useful information the patient is prepared to reveal.

Your first step should be to read the referral letter. During the interview, you will be using a combination of open-ended and closed questions. The former deal in generalisations. Other questions require a more specific response.

The successful interview allows the patient to set the course but the interviewer keeps a steady hand on the tiller and makes adjustments whenever the course seems to veer.

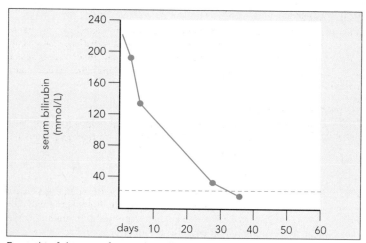

Example of the use of a graph to illustrate changes in bilirubin levels following acute type A hepatitis.

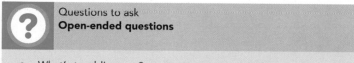

?   Questions to ask
Open-ended questions

- What's troubling you?
- What brought you to see the doctor?
- What brought you to the hospital?
- What are your symptoms?
- The referral letter tells me something of your symptoms but can you describe them to me?

Doctors often overlook the psychodynamic components of a physical illness or fail to recognise that bodily complaints can reflect a primary psychological disorder; the patient's conduct and body language during the interview can tell a great deal about underlying anxieties, neuroses and depression.

THE INTERVIEW

SETTING

If possible, you should find a quiet room in which to conduct the interview. In the outpatient department, arrange the patient's seat close to yours rather than confront them across a desk.

YOURSELF

The patient's first judgment of any doctor or student is based on appearance and therefore dress plays an important role in the doctor–patient relationship. The white coat and personal presentation are part of our medical culture and are important in establishing the 'role-play' that underlies the medical interview.

INITIAL APPROACH

You should introduce yourself, then pull up a chair rather than sit on a patient's bed. Give the patient an outline of what you intend to do and also an idea of how long it may take.

First questions

Begin by asking the patient to outline the problem by using an open-ended question. If the patient has multiple complaints, list them chronologically rather than in the haphazard order patients sometimes offer them. At this stage you will be writing a summary of the patient's comments.

THE HISTORY
History of the presenting complaint(s)

You now need to explore each of the patient's symptoms in greater detail.

There are four fundamental questions requiring answers:

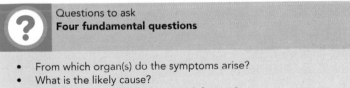

> **?** Questions to ask
> **Four fundamental questions**
>
> - From which organ(s) do the symptoms arise?
> - What is the likely cause?
> - Are there any predisposing or risk factors?
> - Are there any complications?

For each symptom, explore the three items listed in the summary box below:

> Summary
> **Symptoms**
>
> - Mode of onset
> - Static, decreasing or increasing in severity
> - Exacerbating and relieving factors

For the assessment of pain, use the framework shown in the summary box below:

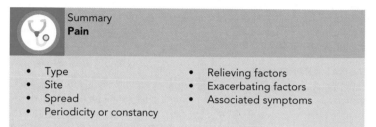

Summary
Pain

- Type
- Site
- Spread
- Periodicity or constancy

- Relieving factors
- Exacerbating factors
- Associated symptoms

SOCIAL HISTORY
Education
Enquire about the age at which the patient left school and whether they attained any form of higher education or vocational skill. This may provide useful background information and, in particular, provide a baseline for assessing any deterioration in intellect.

Employment history
Enquire about working conditions as this may be of critical importance if there is suspicion of exposure to an occupational hazard.

It is useful to enquire about specific stress in the workplace or threats of unemployment.

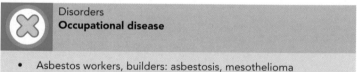

Disorders
Occupational disease

- Asbestos workers, builders: asbestosis, mesothelioma
- Coal miners: coal worker's pneumoconiosis
- Gold, copper and tin miners: silicosis
- Farmers, vets, abbatoir workers: brucellosis
- Aniline dye workers: bladder cancer
- Healthcare professionals: hepatitis B

Drug history
Many patients do not know the names of their medication and it is useful to ask for the labelled bottles or a written medicines list. Remember to ask about nonprescription medicines. Ask about the duration of medicine use. Ask women of reproductive age about their choice of contraceptive and postmenopausal women about hormone replacement therapy. Ask about and list any drug allergies.

Ask the patient about the use of illicit drugs. Your enquiry needs to be sensitively phrased and will be influenced by the patient's age and background

Tobacco consumption
Ask what form of tobacco they consume and for how long they have been smoking.

Alcohol consumption
Unlike smoking, alcohol history is often inaccurate and the tendency is to underestimate intake. Establish the type of alcohol the patient consumes: many will admit to a preference, making an estimate of consumption more straightforward. Calculate the amount in units.

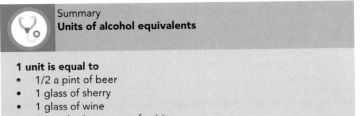

Summary
Units of alcohol equivalents

1 unit is equal to
- 1/2 a pint of beer
- 1 glass of sherry
- 1 glass of wine
- 1 standard measure of spirits

Foreign travel
Ask the patient if they have been abroad recently. If so, determine the countries visited and the levels of hygiene maintained.

Risk factors
Travel-related risks

Viral complaints
- Hepatitis A, B and E
- Yellow fever
- Rabies
- Polio

Parasitic and protozoan diseases
- Malaria
- Schistosomiasis
- Trypanosomiasis
- Amoebiasis

Bacterial complaints
- Salmonella
- Shigella
- Enteropathogenic *Escherichia coli*
- Cholera
- Meningitis
- Tetanus

Home circumstances

At this stage, ascertain how the patient was coping in the community before their illness. The issue is particularly relevant for elderly patients and individuals with poor domestic and social support networks.

FAMILY HISTORY

Although enquiry into the family history may primarily reveal evidence of an inherited disorder, information about the immediate family may have considerable bearing on the patient's symptoms.

Disorders
Common disorders expressed in families

- Hyperlipidaemia (ischaemic heart disease)
- Diabetes mellitus
- Hypertension
- Myopia
- Alcoholism
- Depression
- Osteoporosis
- Cancer (bowel, ovarian, breast)

SYSTEMS REVIEW

Before concentrating on individual systems ask some general questions about the patient's health, this leads in to the systems' enquiry. The questions surrounding the presenting complaint will often have completed the systematic enquiry for that organ and there is no need to repeat questions already asked but simply to indicate 'see above'. Develop a routine that helps to avoid missing out a particular system.

CARDIOVASCULAR SYSTEM
Chest pain
Dyspnoea
Ankle swelling
Palpitations

RESPIRATORY SYSTEM
Cough
Haemoptysis
Wheezing

GASTROINTESTINAL SYSTEM
Change in weight
Abdominal pain
Vomiting
Flatulence and regurgitation
Dysphagia
Bowel habit

GENITOURINARY SYSTEM
Frequency
Pain
Altered bladder control
Menstruation
Sexual activity

NERVOUS SYSTEM
Headache
Loss of consciousness
Dizziness and vertigo
Speech and related functions
Memory

CRANIAL NERVE SYMPTOMS
Vision
Diplopia
Facial numbness
Deafness
Dysphagia
Limb motor or sensory symptoms
Loss of coordination

ENDOCRINE HISTORY

MUSCULOSKELETAL SYSTEM

SKIN

PARTICULAR PROBLEMS
The patient with depression or dementia

The hostile patient
If a patient is hostile to your attempts to take a history, back off with dignity but use the experience to try and analyse the reasons for the reaction. If the hostility persists, then terminate the interview and discuss the problem with one of the medical staff.

Examination of elderly people
History taking

There are special problems when recording a history from elderly patients. Consider the following:

Hearing loss: This is a common problem in old age. Patients may be helped by a hearing aid but it is important to speak clearly and slowly, to face the patient, to avoid extraneous sounds and, if necessary, to write questions in bold type.

Visual handicap: Cataracts, glaucoma and macular degeneration are common in elderly people. Ensure the consulting room is well lit and, when necessary, ensure the patient has a helper to move them in and out of the consulting and examination area.

Dementia: This syndrome often becomes evident when extracting a history from someone who appears physically fit. Forgetfulness, repetition and inappropriate answers characterise the responses and an accompanying relation or carer is usually the prime source of information.

Important aspects of a history from elderly patients include:

- State of the domestic environment and general living conditions
- Provision of community and social services
- Family support structures
- Economic status and pension provision
- Mobility (at home and in the local environment)
- Detailed drug history and compliance
- Provision of laundry services
- Legal will

2. The General Examination

The general examination permits you to obtain an overview of the general state of health of a patient and provides an opportunity to examine systems that do not fall neatly into a regional examination. For the patient, the general examination is also a gentle introduction to the more intense systems examination to follow.

FIRST IMPRESSIONS

At this first encounter, even before you initiate the history, decide whether the patient looks well or not and whether there is any striking physical abnormality. Observe the gait and character of their stride. On first contact with the patient, you may be struck by an unusual physical stature.

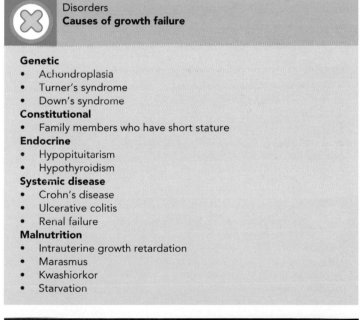

Disorders
Causes of growth failure

Genetic
- Achondroplasia
- Turner's syndrome
- Down's syndrome

Constitutional
- Family members who have short stature

Endocrine
- Hypopituitarism
- Hypothyroidism

Systemic disease
- Crohn's disease
- Ulcerative colitis
- Renal failure

Malnutrition
- Intrauterine growth retardation
- Marasmus
- Kwashiorkor
- Starvation

FORMAL EXAMINATION

Explain the necessity of undertaking a full physical examination. The examination adds information to the clinical database and a thorough examination provides considerable reassurance to the patient.

Begin with a global inspection of overall appearance.

Summary
Observation of general appearance

- Does the patient look comfortable or distressed?
- Is the patient well or ill?
- Is there a recognisable syndrome?
- Is the patient well nourished?
- Is the patient well hydrated?

RECOGNISABLE SYNDROMES AND FACIES

Certain diseases are readily identified by a distinctive combination of physical characteristics. There are a large number of recognisable congenital syndromes that were probably diagnosed during childhood and should not present as an undiagnosed problem to physicians caring for teenagers or adults.

Summary
Clinical features of Down's syndrome (Trisomy 21)

- Facies – oblique orbital fissures, epicanthic folds, small ears, flat nasal bridge, protruding tongue, Brushfield's spots on iris
- Short stature
- Hands – single palmar crease, curved little finger, short hands
- Heart disease (endocardial cushion defects)
- Gap between first and second toes
- Educationally subnormal

Summary
Clinical features of Turner's syndrome (XO karyotype)

- Failure of sexual development
- Short stature
- Facies – micrognathia (small chin), low set ears, fish-like mouth, epicanthic folds
- Short, webbed neck with low hairline, widely spaced nipples (shield-shaped chest)
- Heart disease (coarctation)
- Short fourth metacarpal or metatarsal
- Abnormally wide carrying angle of the elbow

Summary
Clinical features of Marfan's syndrome

- Armspan greater than height
- Above average crown to heel height
- Long slender fingers
- Hyperextensible joints
- Kyphoscoliosis and anterior chest wall deformity
- High-arched palate
- Aortic incompetence and dissecting aortic aneurysms
- Subluxation or dislocation of the lens

Summary
**Clinical features of oculocutaneous albinism
(autosomal recessive)**

- Hypomelanosis or amelanosis of skin
- White hair
- Photophobia, nystagmus
- Hypopigmented fundus and translucent iris

Summary
**Clinical features of Peutz–Jeghers syndrome
(autosomal dominant)**

- Pigmented macules (1–5 mm in diameter)
- Occur in profusion on lips, buccal mucosa and fingers
- Gastric, small intestinal and colonic hamartomatous polyps
  that sometimes give rise to abdominal pain, bleeding and

Summary
**Clinical features of familial hypercholesterolaemia
(autosomal dominant)**

- Xanthelasmas, skin xanthomas
- Tendon xanthomas
- Arcus senilis
- Marked artherosclerosis
- Ischaemic heart disease, peripheral vascular disease

Summary
Clinical features of tuberous sclerosis (Bourneville's disease, autosomal dominant chromosome 9)

- Epilepsy
- Mental deficiency (in 67%)
- Skin lesions (facial adenoma sebaceum, Shagreen patch, fibromas near toenails and eyebrows)
- Flecks of white hair
- Retinal haemorrhages

Summary
Clinical features of Waardenberg's syndrome (autosomal dominant)

- Cochlear deafness
- Frontal white lock of hair
- Wide set eyes
- Different coloured irises
- White eyelashes
- Piebaldism

ENDOCRINE SYNDROMES

The endocrine glands are scattered throughout the body. Both over- and underactivity of the endocrine glands can be suspected from the patient's facies, body build and skin colour; endocrinopathies are often readily recognised in the course of the general examination.

CLINICAL EXAMINATION OF THE THYROID GLAND AND FUNCTION

Like any other organ, the thyroid examination relies on inspection, palpation, percussion and auscultation. Examine the thyroid gland with the patient sitting forward in bed or seated in a chair.

Inspect the thyroid from the front of the neck. The normal thyroid gland is neither visible nor palpable. An enlarged thyroid (known as a goitre) is seen as a fullness on either side of the trachea below the cricoid cartilage or as a distinct, enlarged, nodular organ with one or both lobes easily visible. If the lobes are visible, determine whether they look symmetrical or irregular. Ask the patient to sip a little water and hold it in the mouth. When you give the instruction to swallow, watch for the characteristic upward movement of the goitre as the pharyngeal muscles contract.

Feel the front of the neck for the thyroid gland. Position yourself to the right and slightly behind the patient. Feel for the left and right lobes with the finger pulps of both hands. Assess the texture (hard or soft, single or multiple nodules), symmetry and extent of the goitre.

In the course of thyroid palpation, again ask the patient to take a sip of water and to swallow when you indicate. As the patient gulps you should feel the goitre move beneath your fingers. Complete the palpation by feeling for the carotids which may be encased by a malignant thyroid gland. Thyroid carcinoma may spread to local neck lymph nodes, so it is important to conclude the palpation by checking for palpable regional lymph nodes.

Retrosternal extension can be assessed by percussing over the manubrium and upper sternum. Normally, this area resonates, yet when there is retrosternal enlargement the percussion note is dull. Auscultate the gland for bruits by applying the diaphragm of the stethoscope to each lobe in turn.

CLINICAL ASSESSMENT OF THYROID FUNCTION

HYPERTHYROIDISM

Hyperthyroidism occurs most commonly in young women with smooth diffuse goitres (Graves' disease).

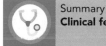

Summary
Clinical features of hyperthyroidism

- Weight loss, increased appetite
- Recent onset of heat intolerance
- Agitation, nervousness
- Hot, sweaty palms
- Fine peripheral tremor
- Bounding peripheral pulses
- Tachycardia, atrial fibrillation
- Lid retraction and lid lag
- Goitre, with or without overlying bruit
- Brisk tendon reflexes

GRAVES' DISEASE

The facies in Graves' disease is dominated by a staring appearance caused by retraction of the upper eyelid.

Questions to ask
Hyperthyroidism

- Have you lost weight recently?
- Has your appetite changed (e.g. increased)?
- Have you noticed a change in bowel habit (e.g. increased)?
- Have you noticed a recent change in heat tolerance?
- Do you suffer from excessive sweating?
- Does your heart race or palpitate?
- Have you noticed a change in mood?

Summary
Clinical features of hyperthyroidism in Graves' disease and toxic nodular goitre

	Graves' disease	**Nodular goitre**
Sex	Female>>Men	Female = Men
Eye signs	Very common, exophthalmos	Less severe
Goitre	Diffuse, overlying bruit	May be multinodular
Heart	Tachycardia, atrial fibrillation	Also angina, congestive heart failure
Weight	May lose weight	Often profound

Summary
Clinical features of Graves' disease (autoimmune hyperthyroidism)

- Diffuse goitre with audible bruit
- Pretibial myxoedema, finger clubbing
- Onycholysis (Plummer's nails)
- Lid retraction, lid lag
- Proptosis, exophthalmos
- Conjunctival oedema (chemosis)

HYPOTHYROIDISM

Hypothyroidism presents insidiously. The disorder may occur at any age, although it is most common in elderly individuals.

Questions to ask
Hypothyroidism

- Has your weight changed?
- Has your bowel habit changed (e.g. constipation)?
- Is your hair falling out?
- Have you noticed a change in weather preference (e.g. cold intolerance)?
- Has there been a change in your voice (e.g. hoarse)?
- Do you suffer from pain in your hands (e.g. carpal tunnel syndrome)?

Disorders
Causes of hypothyroidism

Congenital
- Congenital absence
- Inborn errors of thyroxine metabolism

Acquired
- Iodine deficiency (endemic goitre)
- Autoimmune thyroiditis (Hashimoto's disease)
- Postradiotherapy for hyperthyroidism
- Postsurgical thyroidectomy
- Antithyroid drugs (e.g. carbimazole)
- Pituitary tumours and granulomas

Summary
Clinical features of hypothyroidism

- Constipation, weight gain
- Hair loss
- Angina pectoris
- Hoarse, croaky voice
- Dry flaky skin
- Balding and loss of eyebrows (beginning laterally)
- Bradycardia
- Xanthelasmas (hyperlipidaemia)
- Goitre (especially with iodine deficiency)
- Effusions (pericardial or pleural)
- Delayed relaxation phase of tendon reflexes
- Carpal tunnel syndrome

HYPERADRENALISM (CUSHING'S SYNDROME)

Excessive glucocorticoids (either endogenous or exogenous) cause a significant change in body appearance which can be readily recognised as Cushing's syndrome.

Disorders
Causes of hyperadrenalism

- Iatrogenic, exogenous steroids
- Bilateral adrenal hyperplasia
- Benign autonomous adrenal adenoma
- Malignant adrenal adenocarcinoma
- Nonmetastatic tumour effect (e.g. lung cancer producing adrenocorticotrophic hormone-like peptide)
- Alcoholism causing pseudo-Cushing's syndrome

Summary
Clinical features of Cushing's syndrome

- Round, moon-shaped, plethoric facies
- Hirsutes
- Acne
- Buffalo hump on neck (fatty deposit)
- Central distribution of fat
- Proximal muscle weakness and wasting
- Hypertension
- Purple skin striae

HYPOADRENALISM AND ADDISON'S DISEASE

In acute adrenal failure, the clinical features may be nonspecific and puzzling.

Disorders
Causes of hypoadrenalism

Acute
- Rapid withdrawal after exogenous steroid treatment
- Failure to increase steroid dose when steroid-dependent patient is subjected to physiological stress
- Septicaemia (especially meningococcal)

Chronic
- Adrenal destruction
- Autoimmune (Addison's disease)
- Tuberculosis

SYNDROMES ASSOCIATED WITH PITUITARY HYPOFUNCTION
Hypopituitarism

 Summary
Clinical features of hypopituitarism

Women
- Amenorrhoea, infertility
- Vaginal atrophy, dyspareunia
- Atrophic breasts
- Loss of axillary and pubic hair

Men
- Loss of libido, impotence, infertility
- Soft atrophic testes and loss of secondary sexual characteristics

- Thyroid stimulating hormone deficiency, mild to moderate hypothyroidism
- Adrenocorticotrophic hormone deficiency
  - weakness
  - postural hypotension
  - pallor
  - hypoglycaemia

SYNDROMES ASSOCIATED WITH OVERPRODUCTION OF PITUITARY HORMONES
Acromegaly

Summary
Clinical features of acromegaly

- Coarse, prominent facial features
- Prognathoid jaw
- Prominent nose and forehead
- Thickened lips and large tongue
- 'Spade-shaped' hands
- Excessive sweating and greasy skin
- Kyphosis
- Hypertension
- Bitemporal hemianopia
- Carpal tunnel syndrome
- Impaired glucose tolerance

Hyperprolactinaemia

Summary
Clinical features of hyperprolactinaemia

Women
- Present earlier
- Galactorrhoea (<30%)
- Infertility
- Menstrual disorders

Men
- Present later
- Galactorrhoea
- Impotence
- Signs of pituitary tumour
- Visual field defects
- Anterior pituitary failure

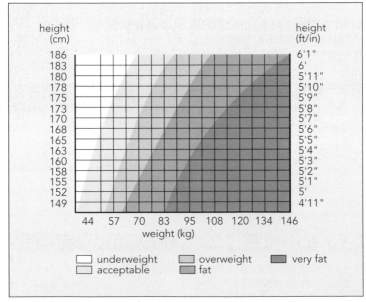

Chart indicating height and weight norms in adults.

NUTRITION

Nutritional status may be an important marker of disease and the progression or regression of a disorder.

ASSESSMENT OF NUTRITION

The clinical assessment of nutritional status includes overall appearance, weight, height, muscle and fat bulk and vitamin, mineral and haematinic status.

Either at the beginning or conclusion of the first examination, you should weigh the patient and measure their height. This provides useful baseline information, as standard growth charts are available to help you judge whether the patient falls within the normal range of weight for height. Ask the patient to extend the arms and hands fully and measure the distance between the tips of the middle fingers. This distance should equal the linear height.

MIDARM MUSCLE CIRCUMFERENCE

This measurement provides an estimate of muscle and fat status.

TRICEPS SKINFOLD THICKNESS

This fold of skin and subcutaneous tissue (the fatfold) provides an indirect assessment of fat stores.

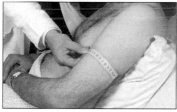

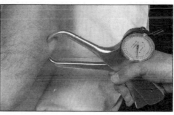

Measurement of the midarm muscle circumference.

Measurement of the triceps skinfold thickness.

CLINICAL ASSESSMENT OF VITAMIN STATUS

Reduced dietary intake of vitamins may result in recognisable deficiency syndromes.

CLINICAL ASSESSMENT OF HYDRATION

Ask the patient whether they feel abnormally thirsty and whether they have noticed a dry, parched mouth. Inspect the tongue and note whether the mucosa is wet and glistening. Touching the tongue may help you assess its moistness. Look at the eyes which should have a glistening, shiny appearance;

Summary
Clinical manifestations of water soluble vitamin deficiency

B1 (thiamine)
- Wet beriberi
  — Peripheral vasodilatation
  — High output cardiac failure
  — Oedema
- Dry beriberi
  — Sensory and motor peripheral neuropathy
- Wernicke's encephalopathy
  — Ataxia, nystagmus, lateral rectus palsy
  — Altered mental state
- Korsakoff's psychosis
  — Retrograde amnesia impaired learning
  — Confabulation

B2 (riboflavin)
- Inflamed oral mucous membranes
- Angular stomatitis
- Glossitis, normocytic anaemia

B3 (niacin)
- Pellagra
- Dermatitis (photosensitive)
- Diarrhoea
- Dementia

B6 (pyridoxine)
- Peripheral neuropathy
- Sideroblastic anaemia

B12
- Megaloblastic, macrocytic anaemia
- Glossitis
- Subacute combined degeneration of the cord

Folic acid
- Megaloblastic, macrocytic anaemia
- Glossitis

C
- Scurvy
  — Perifollicular haemorrhage
  — Bleeding gums, skin purpura
  — Bleeding into muscles and joints
- Anaemia
- Osteoporosis

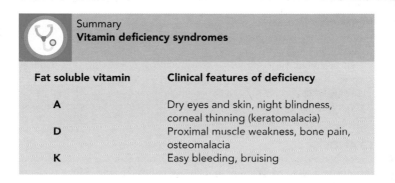

Summary	
Vitamin deficiency syndromes	
Fat soluble vitamin	**Clinical features of deficiency**
A	Dry eyes and skin, night blindness, corneal thinning (keratomalacia)
D	Proximal muscle weakness, bone pain, osteomalacia
K	Easy bleeding, bruising

this sparkle is lost as dehydration develops. With moderate dehydration, the eyes may appear sunken into the orbits, the pulse rate may increase to compensate for intravascular volume loss, blood pressure may drop and the patient may experience symptoms of postural hypotension.

With marked dehydration skin turgor is lost. This can be demonstrated by gently pinching a fold of skin on the neck or anterior chest wall, holding the fold for a few moments and letting it go. Well-hydrated skin immediately springs back to its original position, whereas in dehydration, the skinfold only slowly returns back to normal.

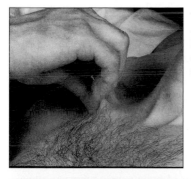

To test for moderate to severe dehydration, assess skin turgor by lifting the skin, pinching it and observing the rate at which it springs back to its normal position.

COLOUR

Once you have assessed nutrition and hydration, look at the patient's 'colour'.

PALLOR

The cardinal sign of anaemia is pallor. Inspect the palpebral conjunctiva by gently everting the lower eyelid. The palpebral conjunctiva is normally a healthy red colour but, in anaemia, it appears a pale pink.

PLETHORA

Facial plethora is usually caused by an abnormally high haemoglobin concentration (polycythaemia).

The plethora causes a bloated facial appearance and, together with the cyanosis, these patients have a typical 'blue bloater' appearance.

The conjunctiva has a characteristic 'plum' colour and on fundoscopy the increased blood viscosity causes the venules to assume a thickened 'sausage-shaped' appearance.

CYANOSIS

Cyanosis refers to a bluish or purplish discoloration of the skin or mucous membranes caused by excessive amounts of reduced haemoglobin in blood.

In peripheral cyanosis, the extremities are cyanosed but the tongue retains a healthy pink colour.

JAUNDICE

Skin pigmentation influences the ease with which jaundice can be detected. The yellow discoloration is most easily recognised in fair-skinned individuals and is more difficult to detect in darkly pigmented patients. Bilirubin has a high affinity for elastic tissue. This, together with the sclera's white colour, makes the sclera the most sensitive area for looking for the yellow discoloration of jaundice.

Expose the sclera by gently holding down the lower lid and asking the patient to look upwards. Eating large amounts of carrots or other carotene-containing vegetables or substances causes carotenaemia which can be confused with jaundice. The yellow discoloration is prominent in the face, palms and soles; in contrast to jaundice, the sclera remains white.

PIGMENTATION

Sunburn is the most common cause of increased pigmentation and this should be readily distinguished from the history. In iron overload (haemochromatosis), the skin colour may appear slate grey. A silver–grey colour develops in silver poisoning (argyria). In chronic cholestasis (e.g. primary biliary cirrhosis), skin hyperpigmentation may develop. A marked increase in pigmentation occurs after bilateral adrenalectomy for adrenal hyperplasia. This condition (Nelson's syndrome) is caused by unopposed pituitary stimulation. Addison's disease may also be associated with deepening pigmentation.

OEDEMA

SYMPTOMS OF OEDEMA

If oedema is generalised, patients may notice tight fitting shoes, frank swelling of the legs or an unexplained increase in weight. There may be associated symptoms linked to underlying diseases such as heart failure and liver, kidney, bowel or nutritional disease. Localised oedema may be obvious if there is venous thrombosis, regional lymphatic obstruction or a painful, inflamed area of swelling. Fluid accumulation in the pleural space (hydrothorax or pleural effusion) may cause breathlessness. Ascites may be noticed as an increase in girth, weight gain or eversion of the umbilicus.

SIGNS OF OEDEMA

You may notice a skin impression made by tight-fitting socks. In long-standing oedema, the skin may become shiny, thin, and even ulcerated due to poor local tissue circulation.

Palpation is, however, a sensitive test for oedema. Press the ball of your thumb or the tips of your index and middle fingers into the posterior malleolar space and maintain moderate pressure for a few seconds. The skin has a 'boggy' feel. The extrinsic pressure will squeeze oedema fluid away from the pressure point. On removing your thumb or fingers, the finger impression remains imprinted in the skin for a short while before fading as the oedema redistributes.

In the recumbent posture, oedema is less obvious around the ankles and most prominent over the sacrum and lower back.

Lymphatic oedema has a high protein content and the oedema is localised to the area drained by the lymphatics. The swelling is pronounced and on palpation the skin has an indurated, thickened feel. This 'brawny' oedema is the clinical hallmark of lymphoedema.

Ascites is characterised by abdominal distention (especially in the flanks) and, on examination, there is shifting dullness.

TEMPERATURE AND FEVER

NORMAL TEMPERATURE

Temperature depends on the site of measurement. The mouth, rectum and axilla are common sites. 'Normal' oral temperature is usually considered to be 37°C. Rectal temperature is 0.5°C higher than the mouth and the axilla 0.5°C lower. Remember that 'normal' temperature is not set at a precise level and there are small variations between individuals (which may range from 35.8 to 37.1°C). There is also a distinct diurnal variation: oral temperature is usually about 37°C on waking in the morning rising to a daytime peak between 6.00 and 10.00 p.m. and falling to a low point between 2.00 and 4.00 a.m. In menstruating women, ovulation is accompanied by a 0.5°C increase in body temperature.

FEVER

Fever may be caused by microbes, immunological reactions, hormones (e.g. thyroxine and progesterone), inability to lose heat (e.g. absence of sweat glands and scaling of the skin [icthyosis]), drugs (e.g. penicillin and quinidine) and malignancy (e.g. Hodgkin's disease and hypernephroma).

CHILLS AND RIGORS

High fever may be accompanied by a subjective sensation of chill which may be accompanied by goose pimples, shivering and chattering of the teeth.

When shivering is extreme, the presentation is dominated by rigors.

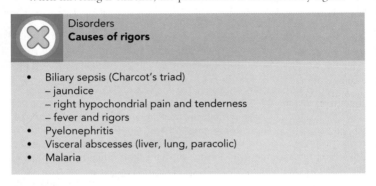

Disorders
Causes of rigors

- Biliary sepsis (Charcot's triad)
  - jaundice
  - right hypochondrial pain and tenderness
  - fever and rigors
- Pyelonephritis
- Visceral abscesses (liver, lung, paracolic)
- Malaria

HYPOTHERMIA

Hypothermia usually occurs with prolonged exposure to winter cold. Predisposing factors include old age, myxoedema, pituitary dysfunction, Addison's disease and abuse of drugs or alcohol. Patients are pale, the skin feels cold and waxy and the muscles are stiff.

A special low-reading thermometer is required to establish the baseline temperature. The most convenient measuring device is a rectal probe (thermocouple) which provides real-time temperature measurement.

EXAMINATION OF THE LYMPH NODES

Examination of the lymph nodes involves inspection and palpation. Large nodes may be clearly visible on inspection. If nodes are infected they are enlarged and tender (lymphadenitis) and the overlying skin may be red and inflamed. When superficial lymphatic vessels leading to a group of nodes are inflamed (lymphangitis), the channels can be seen as thin red streaks leading from a more distal site of inflammation.

Use your fingertips to palpate the regional nodes. Feel for the node by applying moderate pressure over the region and moving your fingers in an attempt to feel a node or nodes slipping under your fingers. Normal nodes are not palpable. If you feel nodes, assess their size (length and width), consistency (soft, firm, rubbery, hard or craggy), tenderness and mobility to surrounding nodes and tissues. Whenever you discover an enlarged node, inspect the draining area in an attempt to find a source. Painful, tender nodes usually indicate an infected source that may be hidden from obvious view (e.g. infected cracks between toes). Malignant lymph nodes (either primary or secondary) are not usually tender. Malignant nodes vary in size from tiny barely palpable structures to large glands 3–4 cm in size. Malignant lymph nodes may feel unusually firm (often described as 'rubbery') or hard and irregular. Fixation to surrounding tissue is highly suspicious of malignancy. Matted glands may occur in tuberculous lymphadenitis.

Often, in the course of routine examination, you will discover one or more small, mobile, nontender 'pea-sized' lymph nodes. The 'significance' of these 'shotty' nodes may be difficult to assess. Before embarking on a major exercise to diagnose the cause of the lymphadenopathy, it is reasonable to re-examine the node a few weeks later. If there is no change in symptoms and signs or gland size over this period, it is reasonable to consider the node a relic of a previous illness.

On completion of the lymphoreticular examination, it should be clear whether the lymphadenopathy is localised or generalised.

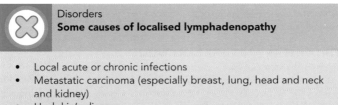

Disorders
Some causes of localised lymphadenopathy

- Local acute or chronic infections
- Metastatic carcinoma (especially breast, lung, head and neck and kidney)
- Hodgkin's disease

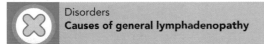

Disorders
Causes of general lymphadenopathy

- Lymphoma
- Acute and chronic lymphatic leukaemia
- Viral infections (HIV/AIDS, infectious mononucleosis, cytomegalovirus)
- Bacterial infections (tuberculosis, brucellosis, syphilis)
- Toxoplasmosis
- Sarcoidosis
- Phenytoin pseudolymphoma, serum sickness
- Autoimmune diseases (systemic lupus erythematosus, rheumatoid arthritis)

HEAD AND NECK NODES

First, examine the nodes encircling the lower face and neck. Sit the patient forward. You may choose to examine these nodes from the front or back. Both left and right sides can be examined simultaneously using the fingers of your left and right hands. Palpate the nodes in sequence starting with the sub-mental group in the midline behind the tip of the mandible. Next, feel for the submandibular nodes midway and along the inner surface of the inferior margin of the mandible. Feel for the tonsillar node at the angle of the jaw, the pre-auricular nodes immediately in front of the ear, the post-auricular nodes over the mastoid process and, finally, the occipital nodes at the base of the skull posteriorly. Follow this examination with palpation of the vertical groups of neck nodes. It may be helpful to flex the patient's neck slightly to relax the strap muscles. Feel for the superficial cervical nodes along the body of sternocleidomastoid. The posterior cervical nodes run along the anterior border of trapezius. The deep cervical chain is difficult to feel as they are deep to the long axis of sternocleidomastoid; explore for these nodes by palpating more firmly through the body of this muscle. Conclude the examination by probing for the supraclavicular nodes which lie in the area bound by the clavicle inferiorly and the lateral border of sternocleidomastoid medially. A palpable left supraclavicular node (Virchow's node) should always alert you to the possibility of stomach cancer.

EPITROCHLEAR AND AXILLARY NODES

To palpate the epitrochlear node, passively flex the patient's relaxed elbow to a right angle. Support this position with one hand while feeling with your fingers for the epitrochlear nodes which lie in a groove above and posterior to the medial condyle of the humerus. The axillary group includes anterior, posterior, central, lateral and brachial nodes. Examine the axillary nodes from the patient's front. The technique for examining this region is described in Chapter 8.

INGUINAL AND LEG NODES

Examine these nodes with the patient lying down. The superficial inguinal nodes run in two chains. Palpate the horizontal chain which runs just below the line of the inguinal ligament and the vertical chain which runs along the saphenous vein. Relax the posterior popliteal fossa by passively flexing the knee. Explore the fossa for enlarged popliteal nodes by wrapping the hands around either side of the knee and exploring the fossa with the fingers of both hands.

Remember that the spleen and liver are important components of the lymphoreticular system. Both may enlarge in lymphoreticular diseases. The examination of these organs is covered in Chapter 6.

Examination of elderly people
Nutrition in elderly people

Many factors contribute to the higher than average risk of malnutrition in elderly people. Socio-economic factors, inability to shop and loneliness combine with physiological changes, such as loss of smell, taste and teeth, to seriously compromise dietary balance. When assessing nutrition in the elderly, the usual criteria are applied. Age-related normal data for height, weight, mid-arm muscle circumference and triceps skinfold thickness are, however, unavailable for elderly people. The assessment of hydration is affected by loss of skin elasticity and the apparent loss of tone can be confused with the cutaneous signs of dehydration. In elderly people, nutrition and hydration are most accurately assessed by a careful dietary assessment (using a third party to validate the information) and use of haematological and biochemical markers.

3. Skin, Nails and Hair

SYMPTOMS OF SKIN DISEASE

The history should evaluate possible precipitating factors and determine whether the skin problem is localised or a manifestation of systemic illness.

> **Questions to ask**
> **Skin history**

- Was the onset sudden or gradual?
- Is the skin itchy or painful?
- Is there any associated discharge (blood or pus)?
- Where is the problem located?
- Have you recently taken any antibiotics or other drugs?
- Have you used any topical medications?
- Were there any preceding systemic symptoms (fever, sore throat, anorexia, vaginal discharge)?
- Have you travelled abroad recently?
- Were you bitten by insects?
- Any possible exposure to industrial or domestic toxins?
- Any possible contact with venereal disease?
- Was there close physical contact with others with skin disorders?
- Any possible exposure to HIV?

> **Disorders**
> **Systemic diseases causing pruritus (itching)**

- Intrahepatic and extrahepatic biliary obstruction (cholestasis)
- Diabetes mellitus
- Polycythaemia rubra vera
- Chronic renal failure
- Lymphoma (especially Hodgkin's disease)

SYMPTOMS OF HAIR DISEASE

HAIR THINNING

Balding (alopecia) worries patients and you will often be asked to assess scalp hair loss. Male pattern baldness is common. Ask about a family history of baldness as male alopecia is an expression of autosomal dominance.

Hair loss may also be a feature of disease and the characteristics of the alopecia may be helpful. Patients complaining of localised alopecia (alopecia areata) may have an autoimmune disease (e.g. Hashimoto's thyroiditis with myxoedema).

Questions to ask
Hair history

- Was the hair loss sudden or gradual?
- Does the loss only occur on the scalp or is the body hair involved as well?
- Is the baldness localised or general, symmetrical or asymmetrical?
- Is there a family history of baldness (especially in men)?
- What drugs have you taken recently?
- Any recent illnesses, stress or trauma?
- Are there other systemic symptoms (e.g. symptoms of hypothyroidism)?

ABNORMAL HAIR GROWTH

Disorders
Causes of hirsutism

- Racial variation in hair distribution
- Hormonal imbalance
  - polycystic ovaries
  - ovarian failure or menopause
  - virilising adrenal tumours
- Drugs
  - phenytoin
  - progestogens
  - anabolic steroids
  - cyclosporin

Questions to ask
Hirsutes

- Is there a family history of hirsutes?
- Are your menstrual periods normal or absent (or scanty)?
- Is there a history of primary or secondary infertility?
- Do you experience visual disturbances or headaches (pituitary disease)?
- What medications do you take (e.g. phenytoin, anabolic steroids, progestogens)?

SYMPTOMS OF NAIL DISEASE

Whereas examination of the nails may be very revealing, nail–related symptoms are usually nonspecific. Patients may relate symptoms suggestive of bacterial infection along the nail edge; these include intense pain, swelling and often a purulent discharge. Complaints of brittleness, splitting or cracking provide little diagnostic information. Ask specifically about skin disease that may affect the nail such as psoriasis, severe eczema, lichen planus or a susceptibility to fungal skin infection.

EXAMINATION OF THE SKIN, NAILS AND HAIR

EXAMINING THE SKIN
When examining the skin, there is a tendency to focus on the local area noticed by the patient. Nonetheless, you should consider the skin as an organ in its own right and, like any other examination, the whole organ should be examined to gain maximum information.

Inspection and palpation
Scan the skin, looking for skin lesions and noting their position and symmetry. Remember to expose hidden areas like the axillae, inner thighs and buttock with its natal cleft. Many skin lesions can be diagnosed by their appearance and localisation. Measurement of the length and breadth of skin lesions is useful, especially when monitoring progression or regression.

SKIN COLOUR
Abnormal skin colour
Generalised changes in skin colour occur in jaundice, iron overload, endocrine disorders and albinism. The yellow tinge of jaundice is best observed in good daylight, appearing initially as yellowing of the sclerae and then as a yellow discoloration on the trunk, arms and legs. Remember that large quantities of carrots or other forms of vitamin A may cause yellow skin

pigmentation (carotenaemia), the absence of scleral discoloration distinguishes this from jaundice.

Iron overload (haemosiderosis and haemochromatosis) causes the skin to turn a slate-grey colour. Addison's disease (autoimmune adrenal destruction) is characterised by darkening of the skin, occurring first in the skin creases of the palms and soles, scars and other skin creases. Striking pigmentation also arises after bilateral adrenalectomy for adrenal hyperplasia: this syndrome (Nelson's syndrome) is caused by unopposed pituitary overstimulation. In hypopituitarism, the skin is soft, pale and wrinkled.

Albinism is an autosomal recessive disorder caused by failure of melanocytes to produce melanin. The skin and hair are white and the eyes are pink because of a lack of pigmentation of the iris (there may also be nystagmus).

Common localised abnormalities of skin pigmentation include vitiligo, café au lait spots, pityriasis versicolor and idiopathic guttate hypomelanosis. Erythema of the skin is caused by capillary dilatation; when pressure is applied the red lesion blanches and reforms. Purpura is the term used for red-purplish lesions of the skin caused by seepage of blood from skin blood vessels. Unlike erythema, these lesions do not blanch with pressure. If the lesions are small (<5 mm) they are called petechiae, whereas larger lesions are purpura. Traumatic bruises are called ecchymoses. Telangiectasia refers to fine blanching vascular lesions caused by superficial capillary dilatation.

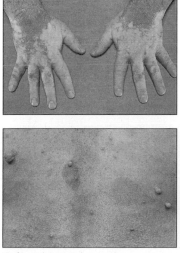

Depigmented skin (vitiligo): white discoloration of brown hand.

Café au lait patches with neurofibromas.

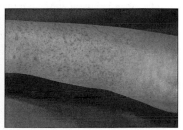

Typical appearance of petechial haemorrhage in a patient with thrombocytopenia.

Localised skin lesions

To establish the primary nature of the skin lesion decide whether the lesion is flat, nodular or fluid-filled. If possible, describe the arrangement of the lesions, that is whether linear, annular (ring-shaped) or clustered. In shingles (herpes zoster), the rash occurs in the distribution of one or more skin dermatomes.

Add to the primary description any secondary characteristics such as superficial erosions, ulceration, crusting, scaling, fissuring, lichenification, atrophy, excoriation, scarring, necrosis or keloid formation.

Palpation is used to decide whether a lesion is flat, raised or tender.

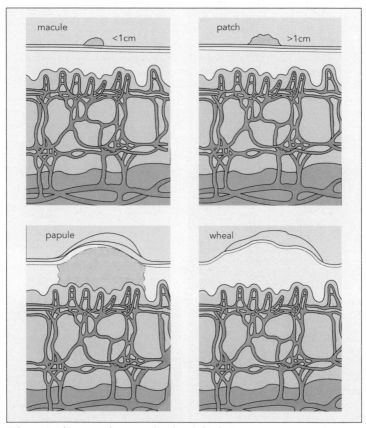

Schematic diagram of primary localised skin lesions.

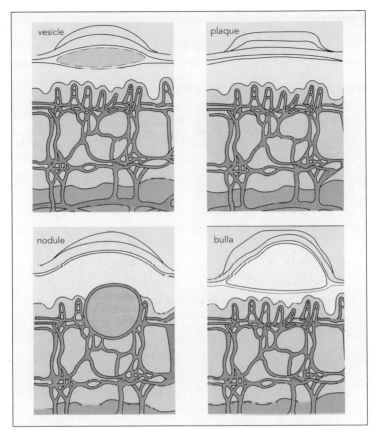

Schematic diagram of primary localised skin lesions (continued).

Compression may be helpful (e.g. demonstration of the characteristic arteriolar dilatation of spider naevi occurring in decompensated liver disease). Use the back of your hand to assess temperature. Inflamed lesions (e.g. cellulitis) are hotter than surrounding tissue, whereas skin overlying a lipoma (subcutaneous fat tumours) is cooler than adjacent tissue.

COMMON SKIN LESIONS
Acne vulgaris
This common disorder of the pilosebaceous unit occurs at puberty. Acne presents with greasy skin, blackheads (comedones), papules, pustules and scars. The disorder affects the face, chest and back. Acne usually subsides in the third decade.

Rosacea

This facial rash usually presents in the fourth decade although, in women, it may present after the menopause. Papules and pustules erupt on the forehead, cheeks, bridge of the nose and chin. Eye involvement is characterised by grittiness, conjunctivitis and even corneal ulceration. There appears to be vasomotor instability and patients flush readily in response to stimuli such as hot drinks, alcohol and spicy foods.

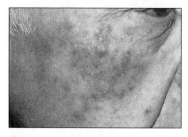

Rosacea: papules and pustules occur on the face.

Drug reactions

Drugs are probably the most common cause of acute skin disease and your history must include a complete history of all drugs the patient may have been exposed to over the preceding month.

 Disorders
Skin lesions associated with drug sensitivity

- Toxic erythema
- Exfoliative dermatitis
- Urticaria
- Angioneuric oedema
- Erythema nodosum
- Erythema multiforme
- Fixed drug eruptions
- Photosensitive drug rashes
- Pemphigus

Toxic erythema

Profuse eruptions affect most of the body. Red macules appear which overlap and coalesce to give the appearance of diffuse erythema. The erythematous skin desquamates as it heals.

Exfoliative dermatitis

Also known as erythroderma, this form of dermatitis is characterised by diffuse erythema and desquamation of the epithelium. If severe, the patient may lose both heat and fluids.

Urticaria

This presents with intense itching and localised swellings of the skin that may occur anywhere on the body. Typically, wheals occur that are red at the margins with paler centres. The characteristic feature of the rash is its tendency to disappear within a few hours.

Erythema nodosum

Symmetrical in distribution, the acute crops of painful, tender, raised red nodules usually affect the extensor surfaces, especially the shins but also the thighs and upper arms. Over 7–10 days, the lesions change colour from bright red through shades of purple to a yellowish area of discoloration. Erythema nodosum is caused by vasculitis, may be recurrent and is most commonly associated with sulphonamides, oral contraceptives and barbiturates.

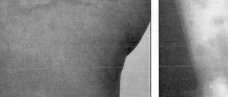
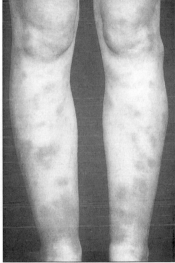

Urticaria: lesions vary in size and shape.

Erythema nodosum: the nodules are raised and tender.

Erythema multiforme

This is characterised by symmetrical, round (annular) lesions occurring especially on the hands and feet but may extend more proximally. Central blistering may occur giving the appearance of 'target' lesions. In severe forms, bullae may appear.

Stevens–Johnson syndrome

A severe blistering form of erythema multiforme with blistering and ulceration affecting the mucous membranes of the mouth and often affecting the eyes and nasal and genital mucosa.

Disorders
Causes of erythema nodosum

Infections
- Streptococcal infections
- Tuberculosis
- Leprosy
- Syphilis
- Deep fungal diseases

Drugs
- Sulphonamides
- Barbiturates
- Oral contraceptives

Systemic diseases
- Sarcoidosis
- Inflammatory bowel disease

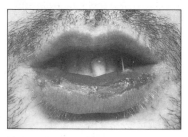

Stevens–Johnson syndrome: ulceration is present on the lips and in the mouth.

Fixed drug eruption
One or more red blotches that may become swollen and even bullous. The rash always recurs in the same anatomical site; usually the mouth, a limb or genital area. The rash fades, leaving an area of skin discoloration.

Photosensitive drug rashes
This rash occurs in sun-exposed areas (face, necklace region and extensor surfaces of limbs). It may appear as erythema, oedema, blistering or an eczematous rash.

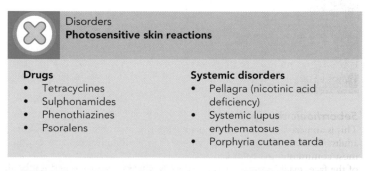

Disorders
Photosensitive skin reactions

Drugs
- Tetracyclines
- Sulphonamides
- Phenothiazines
- Psoralens

Systemic disorders
- Pellagra (nicotinic acid deficiency)
- Systemic lupus erythematosus
- Porphyria cutanea tarda

Eczema

This common skin abnormality is caused by a number of different mechanisms and the disease may be acute, subacute or chronic, all of which may co-exist. Itching is a major symptom. Acute eczema is characterised by oedema, vesicle formation, exudation (weeping) and crusting. In chronic eczema there are dry, scaly, hyperkeratotic patches and thickening and fissuring of the skin. The appearance of eczema is often modified because the patient scratches, causing secondary changes such as excoriation and secondary infection. The boundaries of an area of chronic eczema are less well defined than psoriasis and this may be a helpful sign in the differential diagnosis.

Discoid (nummular) eczema

Unlike other forms of eczema this subtype has a well-defined, coin-shaped (L. nummularius = of money) outline and may be confused with psoriasis. However, nummular eczema tends to occur on the back of the fingers and hands. It also weeps and does not have the characteristic scales typical of psoriasis.

Atopic eczema

This usually presents in infancy. The rash is symmetrical, usually starting on the face and migrating to the trunk and limbs (where it tends to affect the flexures of the elbows, knees, wrists and ankles).

Contact dermatitis

This variant of eczema is caused by an exogenous irritant. Individuals who regularly immerse their hands in water containing detergents or other sensitising substances will present with the rash restricted to the hands. Jewellery may cause an allergic contact dermatitis; nickel is an important sensitising agent. Rubber, dyes, cosmetics and industrial chemicals are common allergens implicated in this immune-mediated form of eczema. Plants such as primulas and chrysanthemums have also been implicated.

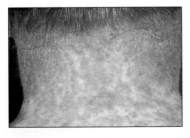

Contact dermatitis caused by shampoo.

Seborrhoeic dermatitis

This is an eczematous condition occurring in infants, adolescents and young adults. There is erythema and scaling with a symmetrical rash. The scalp is most commonly involved. Other regions involved include the central areas of the face, eyelid margins, nasolabial folds, cheeks, eyebrows and forehead.

Pompholyx

This is another variant of eczema affecting the hands and feet. This variant is characterised by the eruption of itchy vesicles, especially on the lateral margins of the fingers and toes, as well as the palms and soles.

Varicose eczema

This subtype occurs in patients with longstanding varicose veins. The eczematous patches affect the lower leg and may or may not be associated with other skin disorders caused by varicose veins, for example, venous ulcers that occur in the region of the medial maleolus, pigmentation and oedema.

Psoriasis

The lesions are well-defined, slightly raised and erythematous. In the chronic phase, silvery scales cover the surface. The lesions vary in size from small (guttate) to large plaques. Guttate (1–3 cm) lesions are widely distributed over the body and may either resolve or persist as chronic psoriasis.

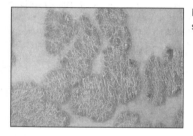

Psoriatic plaque. Note the scaly, shiny surface and the sharp border.

Chronic psoriasis

The plaques of chronic psoriasis have a predeliction for the scalp, elbows, knees, perineum, umbilicus and submammary skin. The lesions are usually symmetrical. A characteristic feature of psoriasis is the development of new psoriatic lesions where the skin is traumatised (the Koebner phenomenon). If you gently scratch the surface of a psoriatic plaque, tiny bleeding points appear.

Pustular psoriasis

Pustular psoriasis is a variant, usually confined to the palms and soles although some are occasionally more diffuse. The pustules, 2–5 mm in diameter, are a yellow colour. On the palms and soles they become pigmented and hyperkeratotic. Rarely, psoriasis may be so extensive that most of the skin is involved and exfoliation occurs.

Psoriatic arthropathy

In psoriatic arthropathy, the distal interphalangeal joints are affected. Large joints may also be affected either singly or symmetrically. Rarely, patients may have sacroileitis or even spinal ankylosis. The nails may be involved even in the absence of skin disease. The typical features include pinpoint pitting of the nail and onycholysis (lifting of the distal nail from the nail bed). Unlike fungal nail lesions, nail psoriasis is symmetrical. Severe nail dystrophy may occur.

Pityriasis rosea

This is a common skin disorder in the younger patient. A single patch rash occurs days or even weeks before the more general eruption. This 'herald patch' may be confused with ringworm. The full blown rash affects the upper arms, trunk and upper thighs ('shirt and shorts' distribution). Pink papules evolve into 1–3 cm itchy oval macules which scale near the edge giving a characteristic appearance. The rash resolves spontaneously within approximately 6 weeks.

Lichen planus

The rash affects both the skin and mucous membranes. It has a predeliction for the volar (front) aspect of the forearm and wrists, the dorsal (back) surface of the hands, the shins, ankles and lower back region. The rash is symmetrical and characterised by small, shiny, purple or violaceous papules which have a polygonal rather than rounded outline. A network of white lines on the surface of the papules are termed Wickham's striae. Eruptions occur after trauma (Koebner phenomenon). The buccal mucous membrane is commonly involved.

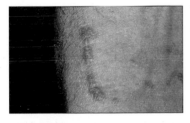

Lichen planus: linear lesion of the Koebner phenomenon.

SKIN INFECTIONS

BACTERIAL

Impetigo

This is a highly contagious skin lesion caused by β-haemolytic streptococci. The face is most commonly infected. The lesions start as a papular eruption around the mouth and nose that then evolves into a vesicular eruption and spreads locally. The lesion breaks down to leave a typical honey-coloured crust.

Furuncle (boil)

An infection of a hair follicle.

Erysipelas and cellulitis

Infection of the superficial skin layers by *Streptococcus pyogenes* is termed erysipelas, whereas an infection of the deeper skin layers is called cellulitis.

Syphilis

In primary syphilis, a painless ulcer with an indurated edge (primary chancre) appears at the site of infection. The secondary rash appears as a pink macular rash on the trunk that becomes papular. In the tertiary stage, granulomas form (gummas).

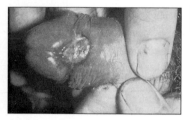

Primary syphilitic chancre on the frenulum.

VIRAL

Warts

Warts usually occur on the fingers and hands as discrete papules with a typical irregular surface.

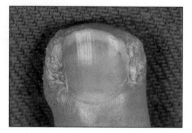

Finger warts.

Molluscum contagiosum

Caused by a member of the poxvirus group. The most characteristic feature of the lesion is umbilication.

Herpes simplex

Type 1 virus normally affects the mouth and lips, whereas type 2 usually affects the genitals.

Herpes zoster (shingles)

After an attack of chicken pox, reactivation of the virus causes a localised eruption called shingles. A crop of vesicles appear in a characteristic dermatomal distribution.

FUNGAL
Candida albicans
Look for candidosis in the mouth; other manifestations include vulval and vaginal infections.

Pityriasis versicolor (tinea versicolor)
Presents as small pigmented or hypopigmented macules on the upper trunk and arms.

Dermatophytes (tinea)
Hair infection (tinea capitis) presents with localised patches of hair loss and skin inflammation. Skin infection (tinea corporis) affects the unhairy parts of the body. Athlete's foot (tinea pedis) appears as a scaling erythematous rash between the toes.

INFESTATIONS
Pediculosis
Infestation with lice causes skin irritation. The diagnosis is made by careful inspection of the hair for eggs (nits) which cannot be shaken off the hair.

Scabies
Consider scabies in any patient presenting with widespread pruritus. The burrows can be seen on inspection; look for these along the sides of the fingers, the webs and the wrist.

BLISTERING LESIONS
Bullous pemphigoid
The lesions appear as tense, mainly symmetrical blisters.

Pemphigus
This autoimmune disorder occurs most commonly in middle-aged Ashkenazi Jews. The lesions often start in the mouth or genital mucous membrane. Patients usually present once the skin is involved. Pemphigus is

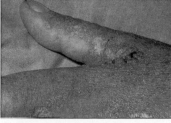

Chronic scabies in the webs between fingers.

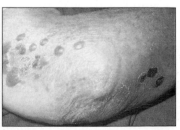

Tense blisters of bullous pemphigoid.

characterised by painful, flaccid blisters that rupture to reveal a raw base that heals slowly.

Dermatitis herpetiformis
This disorder is characterised by strikingly symmetrical groups of intensely itchy vesicles which most commonly erupt on the elbows, below the knees, buttocks, back and scalp.

Naevi
The junctional naevus is a flat or slightly raised smooth lesion. A compound naevus is a raised, rounded, pigmented papular lesion from which hairs may project. Dermal naevi are raised, flesh-coloured, dome-shaped lesions with a wrinkled surface, occurring most commonly on the face.

Café au lait patches
Flat, coffee-coloured patches which may occur as a benign blemish or a marker of neurofibromatosis (Von Recklinghausen's disease).

TUMOURS
Squamous cell carcinoma
Presents as an ulcer or nodule with a firm indurated margin; the ulcer margin is often everted.

Basal cell carcinoma
Like squamous cell carcinoma, sun-exposure is an important predisposing factor. The 'rodent' ulcer starts as a small painless papule which ulcerates.

Malignant melanoma
The tumour is usually pigmented and presents either as a nodule or a spreading area of pigmentation.

Kaposi's sarcoma
This tumour was once restricted to equatorial black Africans and elderly Ashkenazi Jews. Immunosuppression is an important predisposing factor and the sarcoma is particularly associated with AIDS.

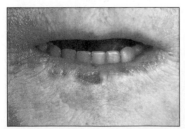
Squamous cell carcinoma of the lip.

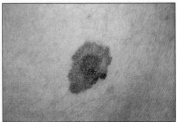
Spreading malignant melanoma.

NAIL DISORDERS

Asymmetrical splinter-like lesions (splinter haemorrhages) may indicate microemboli from infected heart valves (subacute bacterial endocarditis) or vasculitis. Premature lifting of the distal nail is called onycholysis. White nails with loss of the lunule (leukonychia) is typical of hypoalbuminaemia and severe chronic ill health.

Infection of the skin adjacent to the nail is called paronychia. Spooning of the nail (koilonychia) occurs in iron deficiency.

Always examine the lateral outline of the nails and fingertip to check for clubbing. The normal angle between the finger nail and nail base is 160°.

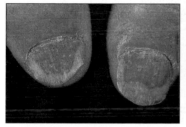

Pitting and onycholysis of the nail caused by psoriasis.

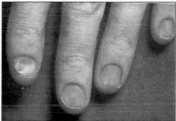

Spooning of the nails.

Leukonychia in a patient with liver disease and hypoalbuminaemia.

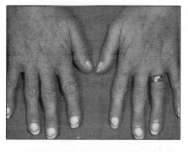

Clubbing. The angle is increased and filled in and the nail base has a spongy consistency.

floating nail base

increased angle (180°)

Disorders
Causes of finger clubbing

Lung disease
- Pyogenic (abscess, bronchiectasis, empyema)
- Bronchogenic carcinoma
- Fibrosing alveolitis

Heart disease
- Cyanotic congenital heart disease

- Subacute bacterial endocarditis

Gastrointestinal disease
- Cirrhosis
- Ulcerative colitis
- Crohn's disease

Idiopathic/congenital

Disorders
Skin manifestations of systemic disease

Disease	Skin findings
Sarcoidosis	Erythema nodosum, lupus pernio, nodules in scars
Scleroderma	Thickened tight skin (especially fingers), skin telangiectasia, calcified skin nodules
Hyperlipidaemia	Xanthelasmata of eyelids, xanthomas of elbows, knuckles, buttock, soles and palms, and Achilles tendon
Diabetes mellitus	Necrobiosis lipoidica – symmetrical plaques on shins with atrophic, yellow appearance and waxy feel; cutaneous candida, ulcers on feet
Hyperthyroidism	Pretibial myxoedema – thickened skin on front of shin, clubbing
Cushing's syndrome	Purple striae, thin skin, easy bruising
Ulcerative colitis/ Crohn's disease	Pyoderma gangrenosum – large ulcer
Dermatomyositis	Oedema and mauve discoloration of eyelid, erythema of the knuckles and other bony parts such as elbow and shoulder tip; photosensitive 'butterfly rash' on face
Cancer	Acanthosis nigricans – brown, velvet-like thickening of skin in axilla and groin; teilosis – thickening of palms/soles; ichthyosis – fish-skin appearance

Examination of elderly people
Skin changes in elderly people

Skin changes are cardinal signs of the ageing process. In elderly people, the skin becomes increasingly wrinkled, representing progressive loss of collagen and elastic tissue and increasingly fragile so that minor trauma results in wounding and secondary infection. Elderly atrophic skin loses elasticity and 'spring' and consequently, assessment of hydration using skin turgor is unreliable. Capillary fragility results in easy intradermal bleeding (senile purpura and ecchymosis) and warty pigmented lesions (senile actinic keratosis) may become widespread. Sun-exposed ageing skin is susceptible to malignant change (basal and squamous cell cancer).

Pressure sores are a major concern in the immobilised elderly patient. Predisposing factors include pressure (causing capillary occlusion), friction and moisture which favours secondary infection. The lesions develop over areas of bony prominence, especially the heels and sacrum.

4. Ear, Nose and Throat

SYMPTOMS OF MOUTH AND THROAT DISORDERS

Patients with disorders arising in the mouth or throat usually complain of pain, a sensation of a lump in the throat, a hoarse voice, difficulty in breathing (upper airway obstruction), difficulty in swallowing (dysphagia), pain on swallowing (odynophagia), a lump in the neck and halitosis (bad breath).

SORE MOUTH OR THROAT

The oral mucosa may be diffusely inflamed in vitamin deficiency states, in fungal infections ('thrush') or after radiotherapy for malignant disease. The presence of diffuse fungal infection should alert you to the possibility of AIDS. Pain arising more posteriorly may be due to tonsillitis or pharyngitis.

Questions to ask
Sore mouth or throat

- How long have you had the pain?
- Does the pain change in severity?
- What aggravates and what relieves the pain?
- Is the pain local or diffuse?
- What other illnesses do you have?
- Are you taking any medication; if so, then what type?
- How much do you smoke a day?
- How much alcohol do you consume in a week?

LUMP IN THE THROAT

Questions to ask
Lump in the throat

- How long have you noticed this sensation?
- Is it getting better or worse?
- Do you have trouble swallowing (dysphagia)?
- Is the act of swallowing painful (odynophagia)?
- Have you experienced any weight loss?
- What factors aggravate and what relieve the pain?
- Do you suffer from heartburn, indigestion, taste of acid in the mouth, that is, symptoms of gastro-oesophageal reflux?

The globus syndrome is described as a sensation or a lump in the throat. The majority of patients have no serious disease and need assurance. A small percentage will have gastro-oesophageal reflux.

HOARSE VOICE

The majority of patients with a hoarse voice have an inflammatory disorder of the larynx (laryngitis). However, any patient with hoarseness that has not resolved after 3 weeks should have the larynx visualised. A history of excessive smoking, alcohol (especially spirits) and poor periodontal and dental hygiene should alert you to the possibility of a malignancy. The causes of hoarseness also vary in different age groups.

Questions to ask
Hoarse voice

- How long has the hoarseness been present?
- Has there been any previous upper respiratory tract infection?
- Have you abused your voice, for example, shouting at sports events or singing at a party or concert?
- Do you smoke; if so, how many a day?
- How much alcohol do you drink?
- What type of work do you do?

Disorders
Likely causes of hoarseness or dysphonia

Neonate	Congenital abnormality
(abnormal cry)	Neurological disorder
Infant	Congenital abnormality
	Neurological disorder
	Inflammation (croup or upper respiratory tract infection [URTI])
Toddler	Inflammation (croup or URTI)
Child	Inflammation (laryngitis)
	Vocal nodules (voice abuse)
Adult	Inflammatory and traumatic laryngitis
	Vocal nodules (voice abuse)
	Dysphonia (voice abuse or misuse)
	Carcinoma

OBSTRUCTED AIRWAY

With upper airway obstruction the patient may point to the throat or neck or describe a feeling of 'tightness' in the throat. The causes of an obstructed upper airway differ according to the age of the patient.

Snoring is also caused by an obstructed airway. The obstruction may be nasal, postnasal (e.g. enlarged adenoid), oropharyngeal (e.g. tonsils, lax palate and fauceal pillars) or laryngeal (e.g. congenital abnormalities in children). If snoring is severe this may be associated with apnoeic episodes during sleep.

> **Disorders**
> **Likely causes of obstructed upper airway**
>
> | Neonate | Congenital abnormality |
> |---------|------------------------|
> | **Infant** | Congenital abnormality |
> | | Inflammation (croup) |
> | **Toddler** | Inflammation (croup or supraglottis) |
> | | Foreign body |
> | | Congenital abnormality |
> | **Child** | Inflammation (croup or supraglottis) |
> | | Foreign body |
> | **Adult** | Inflammatory (supraglottis) |
> | | Carcinoma (usually over 50 years old) |

PAIN ON SWALLOWING

Painful swallowing is called odynophagia. Swallowing is usually painful in the presence of inflammation in the hypopharynx or oesophagus (e.g. candidiasis) but rarely is the presenting complaint in oesophageal carcinoma. These patients usually present initially with dysphagia before the act of swallowing becomes painful.

LUMP IN THE NECK

> **Questions to ask**
> **Lump in the neck**
>
> - How long has the lump been present?
> - Has the lump changed in size?
> - Is the lump painful?
> - Do you sweat at night?
> - Have you lost weight recently?
> - Do you have thyroid problems?
> - Do you have a cough?
> - Is there anything abnormal about your mouth or throat?
> - Are you generally well?

Most neck lumps are due to enlarged lymph nodes, in which case questioning is directed to a potential source of origin. Most neck lumps are painless unless there is associated inflammation or abscess formation.

HALITOSIS

The most common cause of halitosis is probably poor dental and oral hygiene. Paranasal sinus infection with a purulent postnasal discharge may lead to halitosis. Infection of the oral cavity, the gums in particular (gingivitis), may give rise to foul smelling breath.

SYMPTOMS OF NASAL DISORDERS

BLOCKED NOSE

Mechanical abnormalities (e.g. a deviated septum or enlarged turbinates or nasal polyps) will usually cause constant obstruction whereas the nasal cycle and seasonal allergic rhinitis are usually intermittent, the former alternating between left and right sides.

Questions to ask
Blocked nose

- Is the nose blocked constantly or only some of the time (day or night)?
- Does it vary with the seasons?
- Is there any associated nasal discharge?
- Are both nostrils affected or only one?
- What aggravates and what relieves the condition?
- Do you use nose drops?
- Do you sniff glue or illicit substances (e.g. cocaine)?
- Have you had previous nose surgery?
- Do you suffer from asthma?

RUNNY NOSE (RHINORRHOEA)

It is important to ascertain whether there is associated nasal obstruction and whether the discharge is constant or intermittent. The discharge may be watery or mucoid, purulent in the presence of infection or a foreign body and bloodstained in the presence of a tumour or foreign body. In addition, if rhinorrhoea is associated with an itchy nose, sneezing and itchy eyes, a diagnosis of allergic rhinitis can easily be made.

BLEEDING NOSE (EPISTAXIS)

A history of a bleeding disorder is relevant as is a history of previous nasal surgery: septal perforations often crust and bleed. Nose bleeds may be caused by excessive nasal picking or an injury to the nose. Hypertension per se is not a cause of epistaxis but an elevated venous or arterial pressure will prolong any established epistaxis.

NASAL DEFORMITY
Nasal 'deformity' may be traumatic or congenital in origin.

'NONSMELLING' NOSE
There may be a history of head injury. Some patients may report a loss of the sense of smell after an upper respiratory tract infection. Patients with mechanical obstruction of the upper part of the nose (e.g. caused by nasal polyps or mucosal oedema in allergic rhinitis) will also complain of anosmia. In many patients the cause is unknown.

SYMPTOMS OF EAR DISORDERS

PAINFUL EAR (OTALGIA)
Pain in the ear arises from the ear itself or is referred from several other anatomical sites.

Questions to ask
Otalgia

- Where does it hurt?
- Does the pain spread?
- What exacerbates the pain?
- Is there a discharge?
- Have you ever had an ear operation or your ears syringed?
- Do you use cotton buds?
- Have you hurt your ear recently?
- Have you been swimming or on an aeroplane recently?
- Is your hearing ability affected?

DISCHARGING EAR (OTORRHOEA)
Discharge from the ear may contain mucus or pus, and it may be blood-stained. The questions to ask the patient are similar to those asked in cases of earache; the two symptoms, earache and discharge, often co-exist.

HEARING LOSS OR DEAFNESS
The age of onset of the hearing loss is important, as is the suddenness of its onset. The family history is relevant, for syndromal disorders may have some hereditary basis. If hearing loss follows trauma, this may be caused by blood in the external auditory meatus, a perforation of the tympanic membrane or

disruption of the ossicular chain. In addition, the inner ear may have been damaged.

? Questions to ask
Hearing loss

- How long have you noticed a hearing loss?
- Is it partial or complete?
- Are both ears affected or just one?
- Is there a family history of hearing problems?
- Have you had an injury or surgery to your ears?
- Have you had any serious illnesses such as tuberculosis or septicaemia (ototoxic drugs)?
- Have you been exposed to loud noise for any length of time?
- Is there associated vertigo?

✕ Disorders
Likely causes of hearing loss

Infants	Congenital
	Secretory otitis media ('glue ear')
Toddlers and young children	'Glue ear'
	Congenital
	Postinfective (measles, mumps, meningitis)
Teenagers and adolescents	Congenital
	Malingering
	Postinfective
	Noise induced (often temporary in this age group)
20–40 years old	Otosclerosis
	Postinfective
	Noise induced
	Acoustic neuroma
	Ménière's disease
40–60 years old	Otosclerosis
	Noise induced
	Early presbycusis
	Acoustic neuroma
	Ménière's disease
Above 60 years old	Presbycusis
	Noise induced
	Acoustic neuroma

'NOISY' EAR (TINNITUS)

Tinnitus usually presents as buzzing, whistling, hissing, ringing or pulsating in the ear and must be distinguished from complex noises (e.g. voices, music), as these constitute auditory hallucinations, an indication of a psychiatric disorder. Ask questions similar to those asked for patients with a hearing loss. In addition, aspirin overdosage can cause reversible tinnitus.

DEFORMED EAR

Congenital ear deformities include complete or partial absence of the pinna (anotia or microtia). This may be associated with middle and inner ear abnormalities. There may be accessory auricles, often seen just anterior to the tragus or there may be a pre-auricular sinus. The latter may become infected and require excision if it is troublesome.

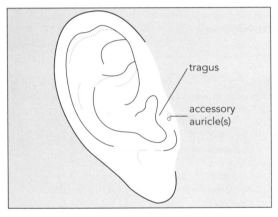

Site of accessory auricles.

tragus

accessory auricle(s)

INJURY TO THE EAR

Injury to the ear may be blunt or sharp. These injuries may result in hearing loss, dizziness and damage to the facial nerve as it passes through the temporal bone.

VERTIGO

Once the symptom of vertigo is verified, establish whether it is of central origin or arising from peripheral receptors (e.g. the vestibule of the inner ear). Central causes of vertigo are more constant and are progressive, whereas vestibular causes tend to be intermittent and paroxysmal (sudden or intensified) and are not usually progressive. However, the symptoms of peripheral causes of vertigo (e.g. the vomiting and the vertigo itself) may be as severe as in central causes.

Questions to ask
Vertigo

- Can you describe the dizziness? N.B. Don't ask leading questions.
- How long does it last?
- Does anything precipitate the attack?
- Is there associated nausea or vomiting?
- Does rapid head movement cause dizziness?
- Is there associated hearing loss or tinnitus?
- Are you on any medication (e.g. hypertensive)?
- Have you ever had ear problems or ear surgery?

FACIAL PAIN

Not all facial pain is caused by sinusitis and not all earache is caused by ear disease.

Questions to ask
Facial pain

- Where does it hurt?
- How long has your face been painful?
- What is the pain like (e.g. throbbing, piercing)?
- What aggravates and what relieves the pain?
- Do you have any dental problems?
- Do you ever have trouble with your jaw or with eating?
- Any ENT disease in the past?
- Do you suffer from migraine headaches?

FACIAL NERVE PALSY

The suddenness of onset and any association with other neurological complaints should be elicited. A history of ear disease is particularly relevant as the facial nerve makes a considerable journey through the temporal bone, crossing the medial wall of the middle ear, the mastoid, before making its exit at the stylomastoid foramen. Questions relating to the function of branches of the facial nerve, such as dry eyes (if the greater superficial petrosal nerve is involved) or altered taste (if the chorda tympani is involved) can give you an idea of the level of nerve disruption.

EXAMINATION OF THE MOUTH AND THROAT

To perform an adequate examination of this system requires certain basic instruments.

Observe the patient's face and facial expression for any immediately obvious abnormalities: these may include lumps and bumps, scars, deformities and facial asymmetry.

Examine the lips for telangiectasia, ulcers, pigmentation and cracks. Ask the patient to open their mouth and inspect the buccal mucosa, gums and teeth. If the patient wears dentures, these should be removed. Note the state of periodontal hygiene and any evidence of gingivitis (inflammation of the gums). Look for ulceration, nodules and pigmentation. Inspect the hard palate for evidence of a cleft-palate or a repaired cleft and for telangiectasia.

Next, examine the tongue and floor of the mouth. Ask the patient to protrude the tongue. Look for ulcers, nodules, furring and leukoplakia (white patches). Ask the patient to say 'aaah'. This will allow you to see the tonsils, the posterior pharyngeal wall and the movement of the soft palate (the 10th cranial nerve is the motor supply).

EXAMINATION OF THE NOSE

First, observe the external appearance of the nose. Second, examine the nasal vestibule.

The nonspecialist should be able to comment on deflection of the nasal septum, the state of inferior turbinates (both size and colour) and identify abnormal lesions (e.g. papillomata and polyps). Assess the nasal airflow. Ask the patient to breath out nasally and observe the resultant moisture on a silver tongue depressor or mirror positioned at the anterior nares. The inspiratory flow can be assessed by occluding the undersurface of one nasal cavity at a time and asking the patient to sniff inwards.

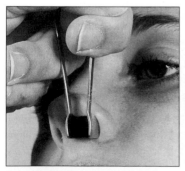

Anterior rhinoscopy using a Thudicum speculum.

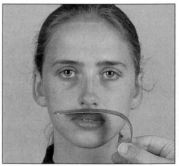

Assessment of nasal airflow on breathing out.

EXAMINATION OF THE EAR

Examine the pinna, note its shape, size and any deformity. Feel for pre-auricular, post-auricular and infra-auricular lymph nodes, again the result of external ear disease, not middle or inner ear disease.

An auroscope with a puffer attached is then used to examine the deep meatus and tympanic membrane. Apply traction in whichever direction serves to straighten the canal, and gently insert the auroscope. It is important to hold the auroscope correctly. This guards against injury, particularly in children, if the patient suddenly moves. Introduce the auroscope and look at the canal wall skin for otitis externa.

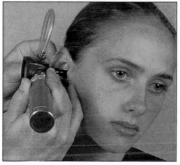

Examination of the ear using an auroscope. Note the position of the right hand against the patient's face.

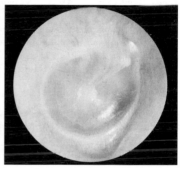

Normal tympanic membrane.

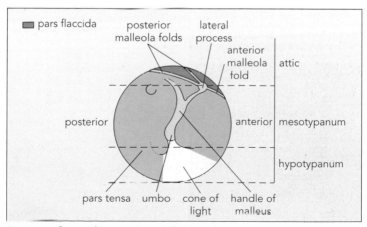

Anatomy of normal tympanic membrane.

The tympanic membrane is inspected next. All the anatomical features of the drum should be actively sought and noted. Note any perforations.

The puffer is used next. This is extremely valuable in assessing mobility of the tympanic membrane; the drum should be seen to move medially then laterally.

The patient's hearing should then be assessed using tuning forks. Tuning forks will give you an idea of whether any hearing loss is conductive or sensorineural and whether one or both ears are affected.

EXAMINATION OF THE NECK AND TEMPOROMANDIBULAR JOINTS

Both these examinations are best performed standing behind the seated patient. The temporomandibular joints are palpated just anterior to the tragus of the ear. The patient is asked to open his or her mouth as the joint is palpated. Feel for clicking or crepitus over the joint and ask the patient if the joint is painful when palpated.

It is useful to palpate the neck in a systematic pattern (e.g. submental triangle, submandibular regions, posterior and anterior triangles). When the patient swallows, locate and assess the thyroid gland and any thyroid or midline neck swellings. The thyroid gland and thyroglossal duct remnants move upwards on swallowing. Cystic swellings of the neck may be transilluminated with a torch. Finally, assess the cervical spine as problems here can present with earache because of the similarity in nerve supply. Active and passive movements of flexion, extension, rotation and lateral flexion should be performed to assess limitation of movement, induction of pain or paraesthesiae in the upper limbs.

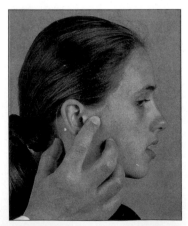

Palpation of the temporomandibular joint.

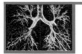

5. Respiratory System

A good history is the basis for a diagnosis of lung disease particularly as examination may be normal even in advanced disease.

SYMPTOMS OF RESPIRATORY DISEASE

The main symptoms of respiratory disease are dyspnoea, cough, sputum, haemoptysis, pain and wheeze.

DYSPNOEA
Patients will express this in different ways as 'shortness of breath', 'can't get my breath' or in terms of functional disability ('can't do the housework').

Causes of breathlessness

> **Disorders**
> **Some causes of breathlessness**
>
> **Control and movement of the chest wall and pleura**
> * Hyperventilation syndrome
> * Hypothalamic lesions
> * Neuromuscular disease
> * Kyphoscoliosis
> * Ankylosing spondylitis
> * Pleural effusion and thickening
> * Bilateral diaphragm paralysis
>
> **Diseases of the lungs**
> * Airways disease
>   – Chronic bronchitis and emphysema
>   – Asthma
>   – Bronchiectasis
>   – Cystic fibrosis
> * Parenchymal disease
>   – Pneumonia
>   – Cryptogenic fibrosing alveolitis
>   – Extrinsic allergic alveolitis
>   – Primary and secondary tumour
>   – Sarcoidosis
>   – Pneumothorax
>   – Pulmonary oedema
> * Reduced blood supply
>   – Pulmonary embolism
>   – Anaemia

Duration of dyspnoea

Disorders
Duration of dyspnoea

Immediate (minutes)
- Pulmonary embolism
- Pneumothorax
- Pulmonary oedema
- Asthma

Short (hours to days)
- Pulmonary oedema
- Pneumonia
- Asthma

- Pleural effusion
- Anaemia

Long (weeks to years)
- Chronic airflow limitation
- Cryptogenic fibrosing alveolitis
- Extrinsic allergic alveolitis
- Anaemia

Variability of dyspnoea

Questions to ask
Dyspnoea

- Is the breathlessness recent or has it been present for some time?
- Is it constant or does it come and go?
- What can't you do because of the breathlessness?
- What makes the breathing worse?
- Does anything make it better?

If asthma is suspected, this can be followed-up by questions on aggravating factors. Follow this up with some more directed questions about particular factors. The house-dust mite is the most common allergen; patients will report worsening of symptoms on sweeping, dusting or making the beds. Exercise, at least in children, is a potent trigger of asthma but exercise will also make other forms of breathlessness worse.

Asthma
Most patients who have asthma are worse if emotionally upset. Nocturnal asthma is very common.

Severity of dyspnoea
Ask the patient in what way their breathlessness restricts their activities: can they go upstairs, go shopping, wash the car or do the garden? If they are troubled with stairs, how many flights can they manage? Do they stop half way up

Questions to ask
Asthma

- Does anything make any difference to the asthma?
- What happens if you are worried or upset?
- Does your chest wake you at night?
- Does cigarette smoke make any difference?
- Do household sprays affect you?
- Have you lost time from work/school?
- What happens when sweeping or dusting the house?
- Does exposure to cats or dogs make any difference?

or at the top? It is important to be certain that any restriction is caused by breathlessness and not some other disability (e.g. an arthritic hip or angina).

Orthopnoea and paroxysmal nocturnal dyspnoea

Orthopnoea is defined as breathlessness lying flat but relieved by sitting up. It is common in patients with severe fixed airways obstruction, as in some chronic bronchitics who may admit to not having slept flat for years. Paroxysmal nocturnal dyspnoea is a feature of pulmonary oedema from left ventricular failure. However, many asthmatics develop bronchoconstriction in the night and wake with wheeze and breathlessness very similar to the symptoms of left ventricular failure.

The hyperventilation syndrome

The initial complaint is often, although not always, of breathlessness. It may be described by the patient as a 'difficulty in breathing in' or an inability to 'fill the bottom of the lungs'. The hyperventilation induces a reduction in the pCO_2, creating a variety of other symptoms: paraesthesiae in the fingers, tingling around the lips, 'dizziness', 'lightheadedness' and sometimes frank tetany.

Dyspnoea and hypoxia

Dyspnoea is a symptom, not a sign. Hyperventilation syndrome and acidosis from diabetic ketosis or renal failure, may produce tachypnoea which may be felt as dyspnoea. To illustrate the distinction between hypoxia and dyspnoea consider that many patients with airflow limitation from chronic bronchitis have hypoxia severe enough to cause right-sided heart failure, yet they have relatively little dyspnoea (blue bloaters). In contrast, some patients with emphysema seem to need to keep their blood gases normal by a heroic effort of breathing (pink puffers); they are very dyspnoeic.

COUGH

Cough results from irritation of receptors either from infection, inflammation, tumour or foreign body. Patients can often localise cough to above the larynx ('a tickle in the throat') or below. Cough from further down the airways is often associated with sputum production (bronchitis, bronchiectasis or pneumonia). Other possibilities are carcinoma, lung fibrosis and increased bronchial responsiveness

An uncommon cause of cough and often overlooked is aspiration into the lungs from gastro-oesophageal reflux or a pharyngeal pouch. Cough will then follow meals or lying down. Prolonged coughing bouts can cause unconsciousness from reduction of venous return from the brain (cough syncope).

SPUTUM

Some patients have difficulty in distinguishing sputum production from gastrointestinal reflux, postnasal drip or saliva. Questions on frequency are most useful in the diagnosis of chronic bronchitis, an epidemiological definition of this is 'sputum production on most days, for 3 consecutive months, for 2 successive years'. Large amounts occur in bronchiectasis and lung abscess and in the rare bronchiolo-alveolar cell carcinoma.

Highly viscous sputum sometimes with plugs is characteristic of asthma.

Questions to ask
Sputum

- What colour is the phlegm?
- How often do you bring it up?
- How much do you bring up?
- Do you have trouble getting it up?

HAEMOPTYSIS

Repeated small haemoptyses every few days over a period of some weeks in a smoker is virtually diagnostic of bronchial carcinoma.

Disorders
Causes of haemoptysis

Common
- Infection including bronchietasis
- Bronchial carcinoma
- Tuberculosis
- Pulmonary embolism and infarction
- No cause found

Uncommon
- Mitral stenosis and left ventricular failure
- Bronchial adenoma
- Idiopathic pulmonary haemosiderosis
- Anticoagulation and blood dyscrasias

PAIN

The characteristic 'pleuritic pain' is sharp, stabbing, worse on deep breathing and coughing and arises from either pleural inflammation or chest wall lesions. The pain may interfere with breathing. Inflammation of the pleura occurs chiefly in pneumonia and pulmonary infarction from pulmonary emboli. Pneumothorax can produce acute transient pleuritic pain.

Most pains from the chest wall are caused by localised muscle strain or rib fractures. These pains are often worse with movement. Bornholm disease is thought to be a viral infection of the intercostal muscles and produces very severe pain. A particular type of chest wall pain is caused by swelling of one or more of the upper costal cartilages (Tietze's syndrome). Severe constant pain usually indicates malignant disease involving the chest wall. Herpes zoster may cause pain in a root distribution round the chest.

Pleural pain is usually localised accurately by the patient, if the pleura overlying the diaphragm is involved pain may be referred either to the abdomen from the costal part of the diaphragm or to the tip of the shoulder from the central part.

WHEEZE AND STRIDOR
Wheeze

Most patients will understand wheeze as a high-pitched whistling sound, that occurs in both inspiration and expiration but is always louder in the latter. It implies airway narrowing and is, therefore, common in asthma and chronic obstructive bronchitis. In asthma, the wheeze is episodic, some asthmatics may have little wheeze and acute severe attacks can be associated with a 'silent chest'. In chronic obstructive bronchitis and emphysema, the associations are less clear cut, with wheeze, shortness of breath, cough and sputum occurring in various proportions.

Stridor

Stridor is a harsh inspiratory and expiratory noise.

OTHER IMPORTANT POINTS IN THE HISTORY
Other body systems

Lung disease can affect the right side of the heart (cor pulmonale). An early manifestation is peripheral oedema (ankle swelling). Disease of the left heart causes pulmonary oedema (orthopnoea, paroxysmal nocturnal dyspnoea, cough and frothy sputum). Weight loss is an important manifestation of lung carcinoma—less well known is chronic airflow limitation, caused by the increased respiratory effort impairing appetite and diverting calories to the respiratory muscles. Gain in weight may be a cause of increased dyspnoea.

Fever generally implies infection, particularly pneumonia or tuberculosis. Less commonly, it is caused by malignancy or connective tissue disease affecting the lungs. If pulmonary embolism is suspected, pain or swelling in the legs suggests a deep venous thrombosis.

Sleep
In the sleep apnoea syndrome, patients are aroused repeatedly in the night from obstruction of the upper airways. The cause is not always clear but obesity and hypertrophied tonsils often contribute.

SOCIAL HISTORY
Smoking
The importance of enquiry about smoking in lung disease can hardly be overemphasised. Smoking is, for practical purposes, the cause of chronic bronchitis and carcinoma of the bronchus. Patients seem to be generally accurate about their tobacco consumption contrasting sometimes with alcohol.

Ask nonsmokers 'have you smoked in the past?'. Risk declines steadily when smoking stops; it takes 10–20 years for the risk of lung cancer to equal that of life-long nonsmokers.

Pets and hobbies
For many asthmatics, cats and dogs are common sources of allergens. Exposure to racing pigeons, budgerigars, parrots and other caged birds can cause extrinsic allergic alveolitis. Acute symptoms are usually seen in pigeon fanciers who, a few hours after cleaning out their birds, develop cough, breathlessness and 'flu-like' symptoms. Parrots and related species transmit the infectious agent of psittacosis, a cause of pneumonia.

Occupation
Any job involving exposure to noxious agents of a respirable size is potentially damaging, the most obvious example is pneumoconiosis in coal miners. In the case of asbestos there can be an interval of 30 years between exposure, say in shipyard work, and the development of asbestosis or mesothelioma.

> ### Disorders
> **Some occupational causes of lung disease**
>
> | Occupation | Agent | Disease |
> |---|---|---|
> | Mining | Coal dust | Pneumoconiosis |
> | Quarrying | Silica dust | Silicosis |
> | Foundry work | Silica dust | Silicosis |
> | Asbestos | Asbestos fibres | Asbestosis |
> | (mining, heating, | | Mesothelioma |
> | building, demolition) | | Lung cancer |
> | Farming | Actinomycetes | Alveolitis |
> | Paint spraying | Isocyanates | Asthma |
> | Plastics manufacture | Isocyanates | Asthma |
> | Soldering | Colophony | Asthma |

Extrinsic allergic alveolitis

Extrinsic allergic alveolitis can be caused by occupation as well as birds. The best example is farmer's lung: the agent is the micro-organism thermophilic actinomycetes contaminating stored damp hay. The story is of shortness of breath, cough and chills a few hours after forking out fodder for cattle in the winter. Other occupations with similar risks are mushroom workers, sugar workers (bagassosis: mouldy sugar cane), malt workers and woodworkers.

FAMILY HISTORY

A family history of asthma and the related conditions of hay fever or eczema are often found. Other diseases that run in the family include cystic fibrosis and α-1-antitrypsin deficiency, a rare cause of emphysema. Tuberculosis is usually passed on within families. Most of the increased incidence of the disease seen in recent years has occurred in conditions of poverty. Enquiry into sexual habits will be necessary as the illness could be a manifestation of AIDS.

DRUG HISTORY

Successful use of bronchodilators and corticosteroids in airways obstruction will indicate asthma. Aspirin and other nonsteroidal anti-inflammatory drugs and β-adrenergic receptor blockers can make asthma worse and angiotensin-converting enzyme inhibitors cause chronic dry cough.

GENERAL EXAMINATION

FIRST IMPRESSIONS

How breathless does the patient appear? If seen in the clinic or office can the patient walk in comfortably and sit down or does the patient struggle to get in? Can the patient carry on a conversation with you or do they break up their sentences?

How breathless is the patient when getting undressed? Is there stridor or wheeze? Is there evidence of weight loss suggesting carcinoma or weight gain from steroid therapy? Does the patient have to sit up to breathe? Is the patient receiving oxygen?

Position the patient comfortably on the bed or couch with enough pillows to support the chest at an angle of approximately 45° and begin the formal examination.

Clubbing

This refers to an increase in the soft tissues of the nail bed and the fingertip. The earliest stage is some softening of the nail bed which can be detected by rocking the nail from side to side on the nail bed. Next, the area becomes flat, even convex in clubbing. This is seen best by viewing the nail from the side against a white background. When normal nails are placed 'back to back' there is usually a diamond-shaped area between them. This is obliterated early in clubbing. In the final stage, the whole tip of the finger becomes rounded (a club). The pathogenesis of clubbing is unknown. There is increased vascularity and tissue fluid and this seems to be under neurogenic control because it can be abolished by vagotomy.

Clubbing is sometimes associated with hypertrophic pulmonary osteoarthropathy; this presents with pain in the joints particularly the wrists, ankles and knees. It is caused by subperiosteal new bone formation which can be seen on a radiograph. The condition is almost invariably associated with clubbing. It is usually associated with a squamous cell carcinoma of the bronchus.

Disorders
Some common causes of clubbing

Pulmonary
- Bronchial carcinoma
- Chronic pulmonary sepsis
  Empyema
  Lung abscess
  Bronchiectasis
  Cystic fibrosis
- Cryptogenic fibrosing alveolitis
- Asbestosis

Cardiac
- Congenital cyanotic heart disease
- Bacterial endocarditis

Other
- Idiopathic/familial
- Cirrhosis
- Ulcerative colitis
- Coeliac disease
- Crohn's disease

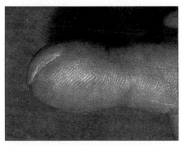
Gross clubbing.

Cyanosis
Cyanosis is a bluish tinge to the skin and mucous membranes. It is thought to become visible when there is approximately 5 g/dl or more of reduced haemoglobin corresponding to a saturation of approximately 85%. Cyanosis can be divided into central and peripheral varieties. Central cyanosis is caused

by disease of the heart or lungs and the blood leaving the left heart is blue. Peripheral cyanosis is caused by decreased circulation and increased extraction of oxygen in the peripheral tissues. Blood leaving the left heart is normal.

Central cyanosis
The best place to look for central cyanosis is the mucous membranes of the lips and tongue. Any severe disease of the heart and lungs will cause central cyanosis but the most common causes are severe airflow limitation, left ventricular failure and pulmonary fibrosis.

Peripheral cyanosis
In peripheral cyanosis the fingers and the toes are blue with normal mucous membranes. The usual cause is reduced circulation to the limbs, as seen in cold weather, Raynaud's phenomenon or peripheral vascular disease. The peripheries are usually also cold. Cyanosis can rarely be caused by the abnormal pigments methaemoglobin and sulphhaemoglobin. Arterial oxygen tension is normal.

Tremors and carbon dioxide retention
The most common tremor in patients with respiratory disease is a fine finger tremor from stimulation of ß receptors in skeletal muscle by bronchodilator drugs. Carbon dioxide retention is seen in severe chronic airflow limitation. Clinically, it can be suspected by a flapping tremor, vasodilation manifested by warm peripheries, bounding pulses, papilloedema and headache.

Pulse and blood pressure
Pulsus paradoxus is a drop in blood pressure on inspiration. A minor degree occurs normally. Major degrees occur in pericardial effusion and constrictive pericarditis but also in severe asthma.

Jugular venous pulse and cor pulmonale
The jugular venous pulse may be raised in cor pulmonale (right-sided heart failure due to lung disease). Other signs are peripheral oedema, hepatomegaly and a left parasternal heave, indicating right ventricular hypertrophy. In severe cases, functional tricuspid regurgitation will lead to a pulsatile liver, large V waves in the jugular venous pulse and a systolic murmur in the tricuspid area.

Superior vena cava obstruction is a common presentation of carcinoma of the bronchus. The tumour compresses the superior vena cava near the point where it enters the right atrium. The resulting high pressure in the superior vena cava causes distension of the neck, fullness and oedema of the face, dilated collateral veins over the upper chest and chemosis or oedema of the conjunctiva. The internal jugular vein is distended amd the external jugular vein should be visible.

Lymphadenopathy

Lymphatics from the lungs drain centrally to the hilum then up the paratracheal chain to the supraclavicular (scalene) or cervical nodes. Chest wall lymphatics, especially from the breasts, drain to the axillae. Lung disease, therefore, rarely involves the axillary nodes. Examination of the cervical chain can be carried out by palpation from the front of the patient. Supraclavicular lymphadenopathy is best detected from behind the patient.

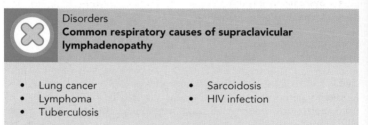

Disorders
Common respiratory causes of supraclavicular lymphadenopathy

- Lung cancer
- Lymphoma
- Tuberculosis

- Sarcoidosis
- HIV infection

Skin

The early stages of sarcoidosis and primary tuberculosis are often accompanied by erythema nodosum; painful red indurated areas usually on the shins, although occasionally more extensive, that fade through bruising. Sarcoidosis can also involve the skin, particularly old scars and tattoos, with nodules and plaques. Lupus pernio is a violaceous swelling of the nose from involvement by sarcoid granuloma.

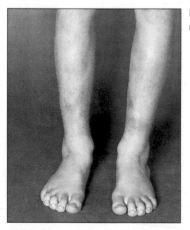

Erythema nodosum, showing raised red lumps on the shins.

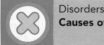

Disorders
Causes of erythema nodosum

Infections
- Streptococci
- Tuberculosis
- Systemic fungal infections
- Leprosy

Others
- Sarcoidosis
- Ulcerative colitis
- Crohn's disease
- Sulphonamides
- Oral contraceptive pill and pregnancy

Eyes

Horner's syndrome (miosis [contraction of the pupil], enophthalmos [backward displacement of the eyeball in the orbit], lack of sweating on the affected side of the face and ptosis [drooping of the upper eyelid]) is usually due to involvement of the sympathetic chain on the posterior chest wall by a bronchial carcinoma

Sarcoidosis and tuberculosis can cause iridocyclitis. Papilloedema can be caused by carbon dioxide retention and cerebral metastases.

EXAMINATION OF THE CHEST

INSPECTION OF THE CHEST WALL

Look for any deformities of the chest wall. In 'barrel chest' the chest wall is held in hyperinflation. The normal 'bucket handle' action of the ribs is converted into a 'pump handle' up and down motion. Barrel chest is seen in states of chronic airflow limitation, with the degree of deformity correlating with its severity.

In pectus excavatum ('funnel chest'), the sternum is depressed: in pectus carinatum ('pigeon chest'), the sternum and costal cartilages project outwards. It may be secondary to severe childhood asthma. Examine the chest wall for any operative scars.

Kyphosis is forward curvature of the spine, scoliosis is a lateral curvature. Both, but scoliosis in particular, can lead to respiratory failure.

Flattening of part of the chest can be due either to underlying lung disease or to scoliosis.

Air in the subcutaneous tissue is termed surgical emphysema, it is as commonly associated with a spontaneous pneumothorax as with trauma to the chest. The tissues of the upper chest and neck are swollen, The tissues have a characteristic crackling sensation on palpation. On auscultation of the precordium, you may hear a curious extra sound in time with the heart (mediastinal crunch).

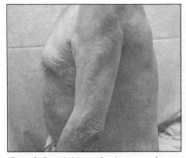

'Barrel chest'. Note the increased anteroposterior diameter of the chest.

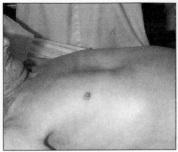

Pectus excavatum, showing the depressed sternum.

Kyphosis.

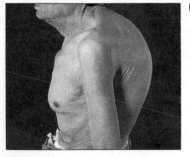

BREATHING PATTERNS

Note rate, depth and regularity. Does the chest move equally on the two sides? Does breathing appear distressing? Is it noisy?

Note an increase in rate or depth. An increase in rate may occur in any severe lung disease and in fever. Patients with hyperventilation may breath both faster and more deeply, patients with acidosis from renal failure, diabetic ketoacidosis and aspirin overdosage will have deep sighing (Kussmaul) respirations as they try to excrete carbon dioxide.

Is the breathing regular? Cheyne–Stokes respiration is a waxing and waning of the respiratory depth over a minute or so from deep respirations to almost no breathing. It is caused by a failure of the central respiratory control to respond adequately to changes in carbon dioxide and is often seen in patients with terminal disease.

Is there any prolongation of expiration? The typical patient with airflow limitation has trouble breathing out. Many of these patients breathe out through pursed lips; this mechanism maintains a higher airway pressure and keeps open the distal airways.

Note if the chest expands unequally. Measure overall expansion with a tape measure. Breathing mainly with the diaphragm suggests chest wall problems (e.g. pleural pain, ankylosing spondylitis).

Is the patient distressed by breathing? Can the patient carry on a normal conversation? Patients with severe respiratory distress use their accessory muscles of respiration. Can the patient lie flat or do they have to be propped up? Patients with breathing difficulty are more comfortable sitting up. Wheeze is often audible to the doctor and implies airflow limitation. Stridor is a harsh, chiefly inspiratory noise and implies obstruction in the central airways. This may be at laryngeal level when the voice is usually hoarse but otherwise implies tracheal or major bronchial obstruction.

'Pink puffers' and 'blue bloaters'

'Blue boaters' are cyanosed from hypoxia and bloated from right-sided heart failure. Carbon dioxide retention is a feature. 'Pink puffers' are not cyanosed and are thin. Investigation shows features associated with emphysema. Cough and sputum are less common, but the patients are breathless. Carbon dioxide levels in the blood are normal or low.

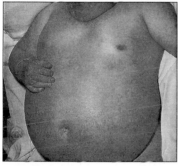

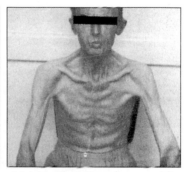

A 'blue bloater' showing ascites from marked cor pulmonale.

A 'pink puffer'. Note the pursed-lip breathing.

PALPATION
Trachea and mediastinum

Start palpation by feeling for the position of the trachea. Place two fingers either side of the trachea and judge whether the distances between it and the sternomastoid tendons are equal. The trachea may be displaced by masses in the neck such as thyroid enlargement. Nonetheless, the trachea gives an indication about the position of the mediastinum. The position of the apex beat also gives information about the position of the mediastinum. The trachea moves with the upper part of the mediastinum, the apex beat with the lower. Large effusions push the position of the apex beat but very large effusions are needed to displace the trachea. Lung collapse and fibrosis pull the mediastinum.

Chest wall

If the patient complains of chest pain, gently palpate the chest for local tenderness. this usually indicates disease of bones, muscles or cartilage.

Disorders
Causes of mediastinal displacement

Away from the lesion
- Pneumothorax
- Effusion (large)

Towards the lesion
- Lung collapse from central airways obstruction
- Localised fibrosis

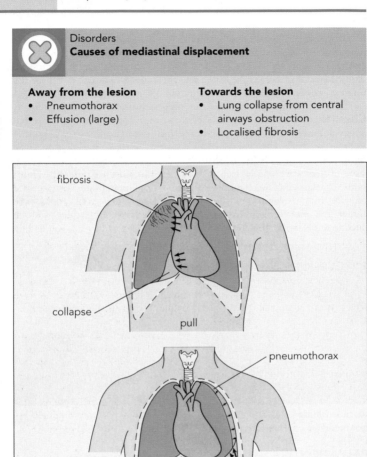

fibrosis

collapse

pull

pneumothorax

effusion fluid

push

Mediastinal displacement.

A SYSTEMATIC APPROACH

Comparison is made between the two sides of the body as abnormality is likely to be confined to one side. Start from the front at the apex of the lung and work downwards. Do not forget the lateral sides and the axillae. Then sit the patient forwards and examine the back. When examining from the back, place the arms of the patient forwards in the lap.

Vocal fremitus

This is performed by placing either the edge or the flat of your hand on the chest and asking the patient to say 'ninety-nine' or count 'one, two, three'. The vibrations are felt by the hand. The alterations in disease are the same as for vocal resonance.

Chest expansion

The purpose of this test is to determine if both sides of the chest move equally. Put the fingers of both your hands as far round the chest as possible and then bring the thumbs together in the midline but keep the thumbs off the chest wall. The patient is asked to take a deep breath in, the chest wall, by moving outwards, moves the fingers outwards and the thumbs are in turn distracted away from the midline. Expansion can be reduced on both sides equally. This is produced by severe airflow limitation, extensive generalised lung fibrosis and chest wall problems (e.g. ankylosing spondylitis). Unilateral reduction is seen in pleural effusion, lung collapse, pneumothorax and pneumonia.

PERCUSSION

The purpose of percussion is to detect the resonance or hollowness of the chest.

As well as hearing the percussion note, vibrations will be felt by your hand on the chest wall. Each side is compared with the equivalent area on the other from top to bottom. Do not forget the sides.

Do not percuss more heavily than is necessary, it gives no more information and can be distressing to patients. The apex of the lung can be examined by tapping directly on the middle of the clavicle. The degree of resonance depends on the thickness of the chest wall and on the amount of air in the structures underlying it.

Patients with overinflated lungs, particularly those with emphysema, have increased resonance. It might be thought that pneumothorax would increase resonance but the difference is often insufficient to identify from percussion alone.

Percussion can also be used to determine movement of the diaphragm because the level of dullness will descend as the patient breathes in (tidal percussion). Dullness is to be expected over the liver which anteriorly reaches as high as the sixth costal cartilage. The right diaphragm is normally higher than the left so expect a slightly higher level of dullness.

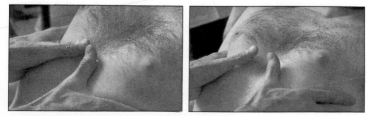

Assessing chest expansion in expiration (left) and inspiration (right).

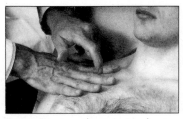
Percussion over the anterior chest.

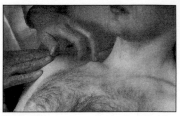
Direct percussion of the clavicles for disease in the lung apices.

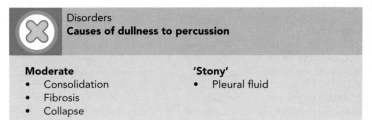

Disorders
Causes of dullness to percussion

Moderate
- Consolidation
- Fibrosis
- Collapse

'Stony'
- Pleural fluid

AUSCULTATION
Ask the patient to take deep breaths through the mouth. Start at the apices and compare each side with the other. The breath sounds are produced in the large airways, transmitted through the airways and then attenuated by the distal lung structure through which they pass. Breath sounds are termed either vesicular or bronchial and the added sounds are divided into crackles, wheezes and rubs.

Vesicular breath sounds
This is the sound heard over normal lungs and is heard on inspiration and the first part of expiration. Reduction in vesicular breath sounds can be expected with airways obstruction as in asthma, emphysema or tumour. The breath sounds can be strikingly reduced in emphysema, particularly over a bulla. Anything interspersed between the lung and the chest wall (air, fluid or pleural thickening) will reduce the breath sounds.

Bronchial breathing
Traditionally, bronchial breathing is described by its timing as occurring in both inspiration and expiration with a gap in between. Forget about the timing and concentrate on the essential feature, the quality of the sound. It can be mimicked by putting the tip of your tongue on the roof of your mouth and breathing in and out through the open mouth. Bronchial breathing is heard when sound generated in the central airways is transmitted more or less unchanged through the lung substance. This occurs when the lung substance

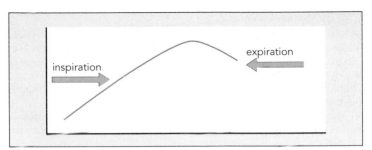

Timing of vesicular breathing.

itself is solid as in consolidation but the air passages remain open. The solid lung conducts the sound better to the lung surface and, hence, to the stethoscope. If the central airways are obstructed by say a carcinoma, then no transmission of sound will take place and no bronchial breathing will occur even though the lung may be solid. An exception is seen in the upper lobes.

The main cause of bronchial breathing is consolidation. Lung abscess, if near the chest wall, can cause bronchial breathing probably because of the consolidation around it. Dense fibrosis is an occasional cause. Breath sounds over an effusion will be diminished but bronchial breathing may be heard over its upper level if the effusion compresses the lung.

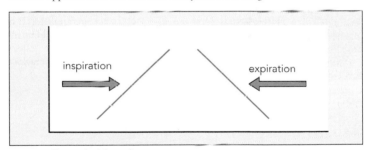

Timing of bronchial breathing.

Vocal resonance

Place the stethoscope on the chest and ask the patient to say 'ninety-nine'. Normally the sound produced is 'fuzzy' and seems to come from the chest piece of the stethoscope. The sound is increased in consolidation and decreased if there is air, fluid or pleural thickening between the lung and the chest wall. The changes of vocal fremitus are the same.

Sometimes the increased transmission of sound is so marked that, even when the patient whispers, the sound is still heard clearly over the affected lung (whispering pectoriloquy). Bronchial breathing and whispering pectoriloquy often occur together.

Added sounds
Wheezes

These are prolonged musical sounds largely occurring on expiration, sometimes on inspiration, and are due to localised narrowing within the bronchial tree. Wheezes are typical of airway narrowing from any cause. Asthma and chronic bronchitis are the most common. Occasionally, wheezing is heard in pulmonary oedema, presumably because of bronchial wall oedema.

Wheeze-like breath sounds can disappear in severe asthma and emphysema because of low rates of airflow. The amount of wheeze is not a good indicator of the degree of airways obstruction.

Stridor

Stridor may be heard better without a stethoscope by putting your ear close to the patient's mouth and asking the patient to breathe in and out. It is a sign of large airway narrowing either in the larynx, trachea or main bronchi.

Crackles

It is possible to distinguish two main types of crackles. The first occurs when there is fluid in the larger bronchi and a coarse bubbling sound can be heard that clears or alters as the secretions causing the sound are shifted on coughing or deep breathing.

The sound of other 'fine' crackles can be imitated by rolling the hairs of your temple together between your fingers. They occur in inspiration and are high-pitched, explosive sounds. Note whether the crackles are localised. This would be expected in pneumonia and mild cases of bronchiectasis. Pulmonary oedema and fibrosing alveolitis typically affect both lung bases equally.

Normal smokers may have a few basal crackles; these often clear with a few deep breaths.

Disorders
Causes of crackles

- Left ventricular failure
- Fibrosing alveolitis
- Extrinsic allergic alveolitis
- Pneumonia
- Bronchiectasis
- Chronic bronchitis
- Asbestosis

Pleural rub

Pleural rub is caused by the inflamed surfaces of the pleura rubbing together. Pleural rubs are usually heard on inspiration and expiration.

Sometimes coarse crackles can sound like rubs; a cough will shift the former. If there is any pain, ask the patient to point to the site of the pain—this often localises the rub. Rubs are heard in pneumonia and pulmonary embolism.

Emergency
Signs of asthma in adults

Signs of acute severe asthma in adults:
- Unable to complete sentences
- Pulse >110 beats/min
- Respirations >25 breaths/min
- Peak flow <50% predicted or best

Signs of life-threatening asthma in adults:
- Silent chest
- Cyanosis
- Bradycardia
- Exhaustion
- Peak flow <33% predicted or best

COMMON PATTERNS OF ABNORMALITY

CONSOLIDATION

Inspection of the chest may show diminished movement on the affected side, palpation shows no shift of the mediastinum but expansion is reduced, vocal fremitus may be increased, percussion note will be moderately impaired, breath sounds will be bronchial over the affected area with whispering pectoriloquy and there may be a pleural rub. Early and late in the disease process there may also be crackles and these may be the only auscultatory change in mild cases. In lobar pneumonia, the changes are localised to a lobe. More widespread changes suggest 'bronchopneumonia', a complication of chronic bronchitis, or 'atypical pneumonia'.

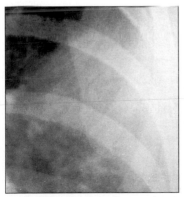

Mediastinum central
Expansion ↓
Percussion note ↓
Breath sounds bronchial
Whispering pectoriloquy
Crackles
Pleural rub

Consolidation. Enlarged view showing air bronchogram.

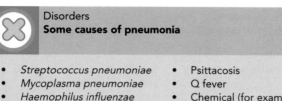

Disorders
Some causes of pneumonia

- *Streptococcus pneumoniae*
- *Mycoplasma pneumoniae*
- *Haemophilus influenzae*
- Influenza virus
- *Legionella pneumophilia*

- Psittacosis
- Q fever
- Chemical (for example, aspiration of vomit)
- Radiation

PLEURAL FLUID

Whether this be from an increase in pleural transudate, pleural exudate from inflammation, blood, pus or lymph, the signs are the same. A large amount of fluid is needed to displace the heart and an even larger amount, filling most of the hemithorax, to displace the trachea. The displacement is away from the fluid. Expansion is diminished on the affected side, vocal fremitus is reduced, percussion note is markedly reduced, 'stony dullness', and breath sounds are absent or markedly reduced. Bronchial breathing may be heard at the upper level of the effusion.

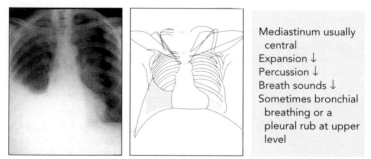

Small effusion.

Mediastinum usually central
Expansion ↓
Percussion ↓
Breath sounds ↓
Sometimes bronchial breathing or a pleural rub at upper level

PNEUMOTHORAX

The pressure in the pleural space is normally negative with respect to atmospheric pressure. In a pneumothorax, the affected side is at a higher pressure, that is, less negative. This pressure tends to displace the mediastinum to the opposite side and if there is a flap valve effect producing a tension pneumothorax, this can be extreme and dangerous. The affected side moves less well, vocal fremitus is reduced and the percussion note is normal. The expected increased resonance can be difficult to detect and it is the conjunction of diminished breath sounds with a normal percussion note that distinguishes it. Vocal resonance is reduced and there are no added sounds.

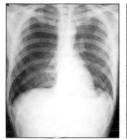 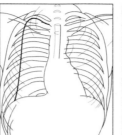

Mediastinum
  sometimes
  displaced
Expansion ↓
Percussion normal
  or ↓
Breath sounds ↓
No added sounds

Pneumothorax on right.

 Disorders
Some causes of pneumothorax

- No cause found
- Apical blebs
- Chronic bronchitis and emphysema
- Staphlococcal pneumonia

- Asthma
- Tuberculosis
- Cystic fibrosis
- Trauma

CHRONIC AIRFLOW LIMITATION

This term covers chronic obstructive bronchitis, emphysema and asthma. There may be hyperinflation of the chest, pursed lip breathing and use of accessory muscles of respiration. Expansion may well be reduced but usually equally so.

Vocal fremitus is normal, percussion is usually normal but there may be increased resonance and reduced hepatic and cardiac dullness. Breath sounds are vesicular and sometimes reduced, presumably from low flow rates; the added sounds are wheezes and often crackles.

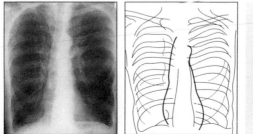

Hyperinflation
Mediastinum central
Hepatic and cardiac
  dullness ↓
Vesicular breath
  sounds
Wheezes and crackles

Chronic airflow limitation. Radiograph often normal but here shows overinflation and flat diaphragms.

LUNG AND LOBAR COLLAPSE

The usual cause is a central bronchial carcinoma, although a foreign body has the same effect. If the lung or lobe is not ventilated, the air within it is absorbed by the blood and the lung collapses. Lung collapse can also follow infection: tuberculosis and bronchiectasis are good examples. Here the airways remain open.

There is diminished movement on the affected side, with the mediastinum deviating to that side. The percussion note is markedly reduced if the whole lung is involved but can be difficult or impossible to detect if only a lobe is involved and has shrunk to a small space. Breath sounds are diminished but remain vesicular in lobar collapse and may be absent if the whole lung is involved. Vocal resonance is decreased. Bronchial breathing, increased vocal resonance and whispering pectoriloquy can be heard in upper lobe collapse because of direct transmission of sound from the trachea.

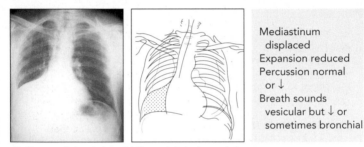

Mediastinum
 displaced
Expansion reduced
Percussion normal
 or ↓
Breath sounds
 vesicular but ↓ or
 sometimes bronchial

Collapse of the right middle and right lower lobes.

LUNG FIBROSIS

Generalised disease is best illustrated by cryptogenic fibrosing alveolitis. The lungs are stiff, expansion may be reduced, but equally, and the mediastinum is central. Vocal fremitus is normal, percussion note is normal or slightly reduced, breath sounds are vesicular although occasionally bronchial, yet there are marked crackles initially confined to the bases but later extending up the chest.

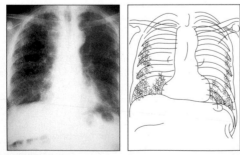

Mediastinum central
Expansion equally ↓
Percussion normal
 or ↓
Breath sounds
 vesicular
 (occasionally
 bronchial)
Crackles

Lung fibrosis.

Examination of elderly people
Respiratory examination

The method of taking a respiratory history and examining the respiratory system in the elderly is not very different from that in younger people. The major difficulty for the student is when the patient has more than one problem which needs identification or when one problem interferes with the assessment of another. Both are more common in older people but, of course, are not confined to them.

Do not neglect an occupational history just because the patient has retired. Asbestosis and mesothelioma can occur decades after exposure. Similarly, the changes of coal workers' pneumoconiosis remain on the chest radiograph for life.

The nature of the respiratory disease that afflict people does not change so very greatly as they grow; one exception is cystic fibrosis. Mistakes are sometimes made by having too rigid a conception of the likely diagnosis in the elderly. There is, for example, a tendency to regard most older breathless patients as having chronic obstructive pulmonary disease with fixed narrowed airways, sometimes on slender evidence. This can lead to therapeutic nihilism. Although it is true that lung function as a whole declines with age, significant airway obstruction is not an inevitable consequence of the ageing process. A history of smoking is as helpful as in younger patients in the diagnosis.

Asthma, on the other hand, is by no means a disease only of the young. Its onset may be in the eighth, ninth decades or even later. Appropriate treatment can be just as effective.

Major problems can occur in trying to distinguish respiratory from cardiac causes of breathlessness and in the elderly both may be present to some degree and need separate assessment and treatment. Right ventricular failure as a consequence of lung disease (cor pulmonale) may be particularly difficult to distinguish from congestive cardiac failure. Both may have a raised jugular venous pulse and peripheral oedema and the basal crackles of left ventricular failure may be confused with those of chronic airway obstruction.

Assessment of disability may be difficult when more than one disease is present. For example, both chronic airflow limitation and intermittant claudication are common in a smoking population; both may limit exercise. Improvement in one may be of little account if the other remains unchanged. Careful assessment is needed to ensure that treatment is well directed.

6. The Heart and Cardiovascular System

The cardiovascular system is fundamental to the functioning of almost every other organ system.

CLINICAL HISTORY

BREATHLESSNESS

Patients with heart disease that causes breathlessness characteristically experience it during physical exertion (exertional dyspnoea) and sometimes when they lie flat in bed (positional dyspnoea or orthopnoea). Sometimes, the patient awakes from sleep extremely breathless and has to sit up gasping for breath. This is often accompanied by a cough and white frothy sputum (paroxysmal nocturnal dyspnoea).

A popular classification of exercise tolerance in heart disease is that proposed by the New York Heart Association which is used widely in clinical trials.

It can sometimes be difficult to decide whether a patient's breathlessness is caused by heart or lung disease. Paroxysmal nocturnal dyspnoea or orthopnoea point towards heart disease and wheezing is a prominent feature of lung disease.

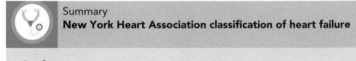

Summary
New York Heart Association classification of heart failure

Grade
I   No symptoms at rest, dyspnoea only on vigorous exertion
II No symptoms at rest, dyspnoea on moderate exertion
III May be mild symptoms at rest, dyspnoea on mild exertion, severe dyspnoea on moderate exertion
IV Significant dyspnoea at rest, severe dyspnoea even on very mild exertion. Patient often bed bound

CHEST PAIN

Chest pain caused by myocardial ischaemia

The single most characteristic feature of angina is chest pain during exertion that goes away again as soon as, or very shortly after, the exertion stops. It is usually described as a crushing, squeezing or constricting pain.

Pain that is similar in nature to angina but comes on at rest may be caused

Questions to ask
Breathlessness

- Do you ever feel short of breath?
- Does this happen on exertion?
- How much can you do before getting breathless?
- Do you ever wake up gasping for breath?
- If so, do you have to sit up or get out of bed?
- How many pillows do you sleep on?
- Do you cough or wheeze when you are short of breath?

Disorders
Differential diagnosis of dyspnoea

- Heart failure
- Ischaemic heart disease (atypical angina)
- Pulmonary embolism
- Lung disease
- Severe anaemia

by unstable angina or myocardial infarction. The pain of myocardial infarction is severe, persistent and often accompanied by nausea and a feeling of impending death.

Pericarditis

Pericarditis may be a complication of myocardial infarction or it may result from a viral or bacterial infection and is usually described as a constant soreness behind the breast bone and that often gets much worse if the patient takes a deep breath. Pericarditic pain is related to movement (e.g. turning over in bed) but not to physical exertion. It sometimes radiates to the tip of the left shoulder.

Disorders
Causes of chest pain on exertion

- Angina caused by coronary atheroma
- Aortic stenosis
- Hypertrophic cardiomyopathy
- 'Anginal syndrome with normal coronary arteries'

Questions to ask
Angina

- Do you get pain in your chest on exertion (e.g. climbing stairs)?
- Whereabouts in the chest do you feel it?
- Is it worse in cold weather?
- Is it worse if you exercise after a big meal?
- Is it bad enough to stop you from exercising?
- Does it go away when you rest?
- Do you ever get similar pain if you get excited or upset?

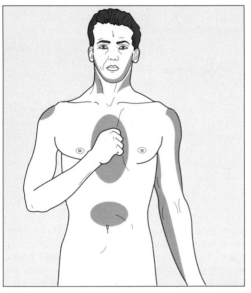

Characteristic distribution of anginal pain.

Summary
Clinical features of anginal pain

- Brought on by physical or emotional exertion
- Relieved by rest
- Usually crushing, squeezing or constricting in nature
- Usually retrosternal
- Often worse after food or in cold winds
- Often relieved by nitrates

Musculoskeletal chest pain

Pain arising in the chest wall or thoracic spine is often mistaken for cardiac pain. It tends to be an aching pain, the onset of which may relate to a particular twist or movement: the pain persists at rest. There is often localised tenderness, particularly over the costal cartilages.

Dissecting aortic aneurysm

Dissecting aneurysm of the thoracic aorta causes a rare but characteristic form of chest pain that usually starts as a 'tearing' sensation, often felt most between the shoulder blades or in the back. The pain is usually severe and persistent and may be mistaken for the pain of myocardial infarction.

Other chest pains

Other chest pains that may masquerade as cardiac pain include the pain of pleurisy, acute pneumothorax or shingles.

Disorders
Causes of chest pain at rest

- Myocardial infarction
- Unstable angina
- Dissecting aortic aneurysm
- Oesophageal pain
- Pericarditis
- Pleuritic pain
- Musculoskeletal pain
- Herpes zoster (shingles)

Palpitation

Palpitation is defined as abnormal awareness of the heart beat. Ectopic beats are often more apparent when the background heart rate is slow (e.g. when the patient lies down to rest); whereas paroxysmal tachycardias are often precipitated by exercise or by particular movements (e.g. stooping or reaching).

Find out whether the arrhythmia is simply a transient inconvenience to the patient or whether the patient has to stop working and lie down. Some arrhythmias cause patients to lose consciousness. Many patients with paroxysmal tachycardia have learnt some trick such as the Valsalva maneouvre which will terminate an attack. In some patients, palpitation is precipitated by tea, coffee, wine and chocolates.

Disorders
Causes of palpitation

- Extrasystoles
- Paroxysmal atrial fibrillation
- Thyrotoxicosis
- Paroxysmal supraventricular tachycardia
- Perimenopausal

Questions to ask
Palpitation

- Please could you tap out on the table the rate you think your heart goes at during an attack?
- Is the heart beat regular or irregular?
- Is there anything that sets attacks off?
- Can you do anything to stop an attack?
- What do you do when you have an attack?
- Are there any foods that seem to make symptoms worse?
- What medicines are you taking?

Syncope (fainting, blackouts)

Syncope is defined as loss of consciousness resulting from a transient failure of blood supply to the brain. The common causes of syncope are simple fainting (vasovagal syncope), its variants such as micturition syncope, postural hypotension, vertebrobasilar insufficiency and cardiac arrhythmias, particularly intermittent heart block.

In fainting, loss of consciousness is seldom abrupt; the patient looks pale or 'green' both before and immediately afterwards. Rapid relief is provided by elevating the legs. In contrast, syncope caused by heart block is often sudden, unheralded and complete. The patient looks pale while collapsed, recovery (which is often equally sudden) may be heralded by a pink flush. Vertebrobasilar insufficiency is common in elderly patients; there may be restricted neck movement, and active or passive movements of the neck may precipitate symptoms. Postural hypotension is more common in elderly people and may be exacerbated by antihypertensive medication.

Claudication

Claudication is the name given to a condition in which the patient experiences pain in one or both legs on walking which eases up when the patient rests.

Questions to ask
Syncope

(Wherever possible, history should be taken from a family member or observer as well as the patient.)
- What were the exact circumstances of the blackout?
- Did you have any warning of the attack?
- How quickly did you recover?
- Did you go pale or red during or after the attack?
- Are you taking any medication?

Intermittent claudication is usually the earliest symptom of narrowing in the arteries supplying the legs. The pain is usually an aching pain felt in the calf, thigh or buttocks.

OCCUPATIONAL AND FAMILY HISTORY

A family history is very important because many cardiac diseases involve an underlying genetic predisposition (e.g. hyperlipidaemia). The patient's occupation may be relevant to the significance of the disease: coronary artery disease or arrhythmias may be incompatible with a continuing career as an airline pilot or truck driver.

Do not forget to enquire specifically about smoking, alcohol intake and any medication.

A FRAMEWORK FOR THE ROUTINE PHYSICAL EXAMINATION OF THE CARDIOVASCULAR SYSTEM

HANDS IN HEART DISEASE

The temperature of the hands gives a guide to the extent of peripheral vasodilatation. Patients in heart failure are usually vasoconstricted and their hands feel cold.

The fingernails may show splinter haemorrhages in subacute infective endocarditis and finger clubbing in endocarditis or cyanotic congenital heart disease.

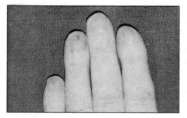

Splinter haemorrhage in the ring finger of a man with infective endocarditis. There is an older, fading 'splinter' under the nail of the index finger. Splinter haemorrhages are often smaller and darker than this.

FEELING THE PERIPHERAL PULSES

The right radial pulse is used to assess heart rate and rhythm, it is not a good pulse from which to assess pulse character. In patients with suspected coarctation of the aorta, feel the radial and the femoral pulse. In coarctation not only is the volume of the femoral pulse diminished but it is also delayed compared with the radial pulse.

Carotid pulse

The carotid pulse is closer to the heart and therefore better for assessing pulse character. Locate the tip of the left thumb against the patient's larynx and then gently but firmly press directly backwards so that the carotid artery is felt against the precervical muscles. In severe aortic stenosis, there is a slow rising carotid pulse. Another sign best appreciated at the carotid is the jerky pulse of hypertrophic cardiomyopathy. This starts normally and then suddenly peters out as the contracting left ventricular outflow tract obstructs ejection.

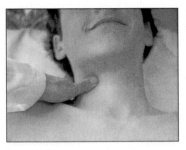

Palpation of the carotid artery using the thumb.

Brachial pulse

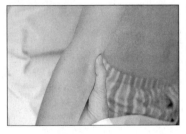

Using the thumb to assess the character of the brachial pulse. The artery lies just medial to the tendinous insertion of the biceps muscle and deep to the fascial insertion of this muscle.

Femoral pulse

It is best examined with the patient lying flat, by placing the thumb or finger directly above the superior pubic ramus and midway between the pubic tubical and anterior superior iliac spine.

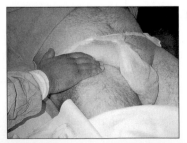

Palpation of the femoral artery.

Popliteal pulse

The patient lies flat with the knee slightly flexed. The fingers of one hand are used to press the tips of the fingers of the other hand into the popliteal fossa to feel the popliteal artery against the back of the knee joint.

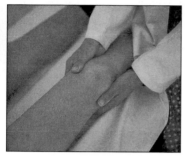

Palpation of the popliteal artery.

Dorsalis pedis and tibialis posterior pulses

The dorsalis pedis pulse is felt with the fingers aligned along the dorsum of the foot lateral to the extensor hallucis longus tendon, the tibialis posterior pulse is felt with the fingers cupped round the ankle just posterior to the medial malleolus.

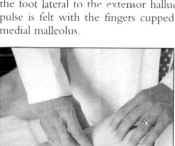

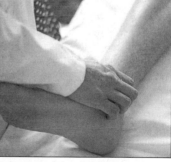

Palpation of the dorsalis pedis pulse.

Palpation of the tibialis posterior pulse.

MEASURING BLOOD PRESSURE

The sphygmomanometer is placed around the upper arm and air is pumped into the cuff. As the pressure in the cuff increases above the systolic pressure in the brachial artery, the artery is compressed and the radial pulse becomes impalpable. As the pressure in the cuff is gradually lowered, blood can force its way past the obstruction for part of the cardiac cycle, creating sounds that can be heard with a stethoscope placed over the brachial artery at the elbow.

Name	Feels like	Associated with
Normal		—
Slow rising		Aortic stenosis
Bisferiens ('two peaks')		Mild aortic stenosis plus reflux
Collapsing		Aortic reflux Persistent ductus arteriosus

Different pulse wave-forms are associated with different cardiac or vascular abnormalities

It is this point of disappearance of the Korotkoff sounds (sometimes called phase 5) which is now used to define diastolic pressure for clinical and epidemiological purposes. In fact, it is the point of muffling of the sounds (phase 4) which corresponds most closely to the diastolic pressure.

Patients with very high blood pressure often have other evidence of hypertensive disease in the form of retinal changes, left ventricular hypertrophy and proteinuria. In patients without these features, it is important not to make a definitive diagnosis of hypertension on the basis of a single casual blood pressure recording. Most authorities would accept a phase 5 diastolic pressure of over 100 mmHg on repeated measurement as defining a hypertensive population. A diastolic pressure of greater than 120 mmHg and evidence of end organ damage would define patients with severe hypertension.

The converse of hypertension is hypotension or low blood pressure.

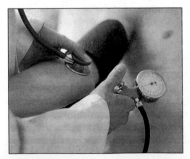

Measuring blood pressure using a sphygmomanometer and stethoscope. The sphygmomanometer cuff is smoothly applied around the unclothed upper arm and the examiner supports the patient's arm at 'heart height'.

Hypotension is usually defined by its consequences (e.g. impaired cerebral or renal function rather than by some arbitrary pressure level). Some patients have postural hypotension, which most commonly manifests itself as dizziness when the patient attempts to stand upright. The diagnosis is made by measuring the blood pressure with the patient lying and standing.

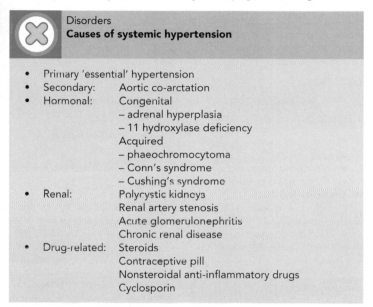

Disorders
Causes of systemic hypertension

- Primary 'essential' hypertension
- Secondary: Aortic co-arctation
- Hormonal: Congenital
             – adrenal hyperplasia
             – 11 hydroxylase deficiency
             Acquired
             – phaeochromocytoma
             – Conn's syndrome
             – Cushing's syndrome
- Renal: Polycystic kidneys
          Renal artery stenosis
          Acute glomerulonephritis
          Chronic renal disease
- Drug-related: Steroids
                 Contraceptive pill
                 Nonsteroidal anti-inflammatory drugs
                 Cyclosporin

Disorders
Causes of hypotension

Impaired cardiac output
- Myocardial infarction
- Pericardial tamponade
- Massive pulmonary embolism
- Acute valve incompetence

Hypovolaemia
- Haemorrhage
- Diabetic pre-coma
- Dehydration from diarrhoea or vomiting

Excessive vasodilation
- Anaphylaxis
- Gram negative septicaemia
- Drugs
- Autonomic failure

EVALUATION OF JUGULAR VENOUS PULSE

The jugular venous pulse is a key factor in assessing the performance of the 'input' side of the heart. The normal pressure in the right atrium is equivalent to that exerted by a column of blood 10–12 cm tall. Therefore, when the patient is standing or sitting upright, the internal jugular vein is collapsed and when the patient is lying flat, it is completely filled. If the patient lies supine at approximately 45°, the point at which jugular venous pulsation becomes visible is usually just above the clavicle; this is the position usually chosen for examination of the jugular venous pulse.

Summary
Distinction between jugular venous and carotid pulses

Venous
- Most rapid movement inward
- Two peaks per cycle (in sinus rhythm)
- Affected by compressing abdomen
- May displace earlobes (if venous pressure raised)

Arterial
- Most rapid movement outward
- One peak per cycle
- Not affected by compressing abdomen
- Never displaces earlobes

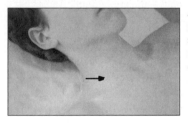

Assessing the jugular venous pressure. With the patient lying supine at 45°, jugular pulsation is normally just visible above the clavicle.

Once the jugular venous pulse has been identified, assess the mean height of pulsation above right atrial level and the wave form of jugular venous pulsation. It is usual to express the height of jugular venous pulsation above the manubriosternal angle. A normal jugular venous pressure is less than 4 cm above the manubriosternal angle.

In patients with a very high jugular venous pressure (e.g. pericardial tamponade or constrictive pericarditis), the internal jugular vein may be completely filled with the patient lying at 45° and it is necessary to sit the patient bolt upright to see the top of the pulsation.

Examples of different jugular pressure wave-forms are shown in the figure on page 97.

Emergency
Severe hypotension (shock)

Emergency medical assessment of the patient with severe hypotension (shock)

1. **History** (from patient, relatives or attendants)
    - Has there been any trauma, haemorrhage or substance abuse?
    - Has onset been sudden or gradual (over hours or days, e.g. diabetic ketoacidosis, dysentry)?
    - Has there been any pain (i) in the chest (myocardial infarction, dissecting aneurysm) or (ii) elsewhere (e.g. headache in meningococcal septicaemia)?
    - Is there any other relevant history (e.g. bed rest, airline travel in massive pulmonary embolism)?

2. **Clinical examination**
    - Before starting the examination, check that the patient's airway is safe and, if possible, attach an ECG monitor.
    - Check whether the patient is more comfortable sitting up (think of pulmonary oedema) or lying flat (think of hypovolaemia or pulmonary embolism).
    - Remove external clothes and conduct a quick but thorough examination for signs of trauma or haemorrhage if appropriate. Usually the skin in shock is pale and cold but if it is warm or red think of septicaemia or allergy.
    - Assess the pulse. Normally it would be fast (100–120 beats/min) in shock, if very slow think of heart block, if more rapid consider an arrhythmia.
    - Quickly assess the major pulses (carotid, femorals). If asymmetrical, think of dissecting aortic aneurysm.
    - Try and assess the jugular venous pressure. A very high jugular venous pressure suggests pulmonary embolism or cardiac tamponade.
    - Check that the trachea is central and that air entry can be heard on both sides of the chest (if not, think of tension pneumothorax). If there are widespread crackles in the lungs, think of pulmonary oedema.
    - Listen to the front of the chest for murmurs or abnormal heart sounds (often very difficult if the heart rate is rapid).
    - Gently palpate the abdomen for tenderness or pulsation (think of ruptured aortic aneurysm).
    - If appropriate consider rectal or vaginal examination for hidden haemorrhage.

Emergency
Severe hypotension (shock) continued

3. **Investigation**
- As soon as possible record an ECG (diagnosis of myocardial infarction, arrhythmia, pulmonary embolism) and take a chest radiograph (and if appropriate other radiographs, for example, in the case of trauma). Consider emergency echocardiography if diagnosis is still in doubt.

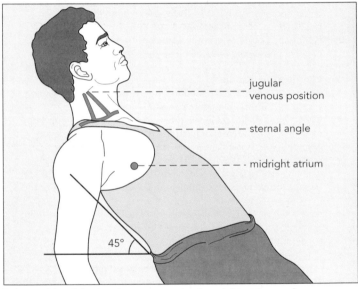

jugular venous position

sternal angle

midright atrium

45°

Relationship of the jugular venous pulsation, right atrium and manubriosternal angle.

Disorders
Causes of raised jugular venous pressure

- Congestive or right-sided heart failure
- Tricuspid reflux
- Pericardial tamponade
- Pulmonary embolism
- Iatrogenic fluid overload
- Superior vena cava obstruction

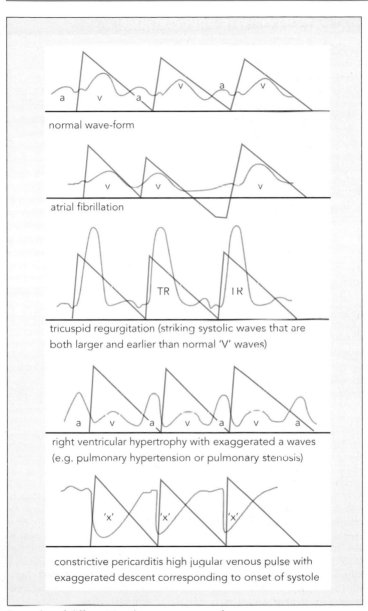

normal wave-form

atrial fibrillation

tricuspid regurgitation (striking systolic waves that are both larger and earlier than normal 'V' waves)

right ventricular hypertrophy with exaggerated a waves (e.g. pulmonary hypertension or pulmonary stenosis)

constrictive pericarditis high jugular venous pulse with exaggerated descent corresponding to onset of systole

Examples of different jugular pressure wave-forms.

PALPATION OF THE PRECORDIUM

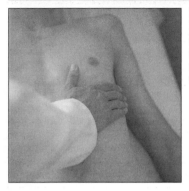

Palpating the precordium. For locating the apex beat, the patient should lay flat on his or her back but to assess the quality of the impulses the patient should be rolled onto the left side.

Locate the 'apex beat'. This is the furthest outward and downward point at which pulsation is easily palpable. The normal adult apex beat with the patient lying supine at 45° is in the fifth or sixth left intercostal space, in the midclavicular line.

Just as important as the position of the apex beat is the quality of the impulse that you feel. A forceful apex beat usually indicates increased cardiac output. A diffuse poorly localised apex beat is found after damage to the ventricular muscle, either by myocardial infarction or as a result of cardiomyopathy.

> ⊗ Disorders
> **Causes of left ventricular hypertrophy**
>
> • Hypertension
> • Aortic stenosis
> • Hypertrophic cardiomyopathy

The character of the cardiac impulse in left ventricular hypertrophy is very distinctive, being a sustained and forceful heave rather than a short sharp impulse. In mitral stenosis, the cardiac apex is described as tapping. To some extent, this is caused by a loud first heart sound which is palpable as well as audible. Right ventricular hypertrophy or dilatation is felt as a heave close to the left sternal order.

While palpating the heart, the examining hand will sometimes detect a vibration or 'thrill'. Thrills are 'palpable murmurs' and are always accompanied by an easily heard murmur on auscultation. Systolic thrills may accompany aortic stenosis, ventricular septal defect or mitral reflux.

AUSCULTATION OF THE HEART

The bell is central for listening to low-pitched sounds such as the mid-diastolic murmur of mitral stenosis or the third heart sound of cardiac failure. In contrast, the diaphragm filters out low-pitched sounds and, therefore, emphasises high-pitched ones. The diaphragm is best for analysing the second heart sound, for ejection and mid-systolic clicks and for the soft but high-pitched early diastolic murmur of aortic regurgitation.

You should listen at the apex, at the base (the part of the heart between the apex and the sternum) and in the aortic and pulmonary areas to the right and left of the sternum, respectively. Relate the auscultatory findings to the cardiac cycle by simultaneously palpating the carotid artery while listening to the heart.

Analyse your oscillatory findings under three headings, namely, first and second heart sounds, murmurs and any additional heart sounds.

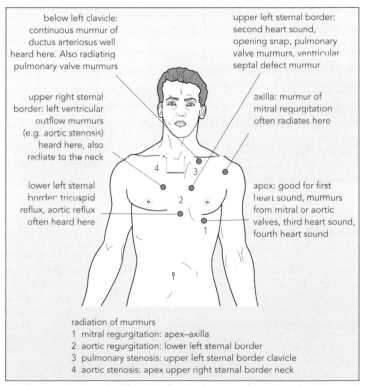

below left clavicle: continuous murmur of ductus arteriosus well heard here. Also radiating pulmonary valve murmurs

upper left sternal border: second heart sound, opening snap, pulmonary valve murmurs, ventricular septal defect murmur

upper right sternal border: left ventricular outflow murmurs (e.g. aortic stenosis) heard here, also radiate to the neck

axilla: murmur of mitral regurgitation often radiates here

lower left sternal border: tricuspid reflux, aortic reflux often heard here

apex: good for first heart sound, murmurs from mitral or aortic valves, third heart sound, fourth heart sound

radiation of murmurs
1 mitral regurgitation: apex–axilla
2 aortic regurgitation: lower left sternal border
3 pulmonary stenosis: upper left sternal border clavicle
4 aortic stenosis: apex upper right sternal border neck

Cardiac auscultation; the best sites for hearing sounds and murmurs depend on where the sound is produced and to where turbulent blood flows radiate.

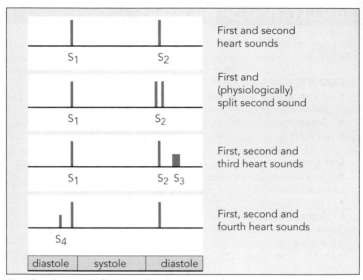

Shorthand notation for recording heart sounds.

HEART SOUNDS
First and second heart sounds
The first heart sound can usually be heard easily with both the bell and the diaphragm but the diaphragm is invaluable for analysing the second heart sound, with the stethoscope usually best placed at the midleft sternal edge. It is usual to record the heart sounds in a shorthand notation.

Factors that may cause a change in the intensity of the heart sounds are shown in the summary box.

Third and fourth heart sounds
The third heart sound is a low-pitched, thudding sound that occurs in diastole and coincides with the end of the rapid phase of ventricular filling. A physiological third heart sound occurs in young fit adults under circumstances of increased cardiac output (e.g. in athletes), it is of no pathological significance. A pathological third heart sound is a marker for severe impairment of left ventricular function. It can be heard in dilated cardiomyopathy, after acute myocardial infarction or in acute massive pulmonary embolism. There is nearly always a tachycardia and the first and second heart sounds are relatively quiet. The cadence of first, second and third heart sounds sounds something like 'da-da-boom' and has been given the name of a gallop rhythm.

A fourth heart sound is an extra heart sound that coincides with atrial contraction. It is usually best heard in patients whose left atrium is hypertrophied (e.g. as a consequence of systemic hypertension or hypertrophic cardiomyopathy). A fourth sound sounds a little like 'da-lub-dup'.

Summary
Factors that may influence the intensity of the heart sounds

Loud first sound
- Hyperdynamic circulation (fever, exercise)
- Mitral stenosis
- Atrial myxoma (rare)

Soft first sound
- Low cardiac output (rest, heart failure)
- Tachycardia
- Severe mitral reflux (caused by destruction of valve)

Variable intensity of first sound
- Atrial fibrillation

- Complete heart block

Loud aortic component of second sound
- Systemic hypertension
- Dilated aortic root

Soft aortic component of second sound
- Calcific aortic stenosis

Loud pulmonary component of second sound
- Pulmonary hypertension

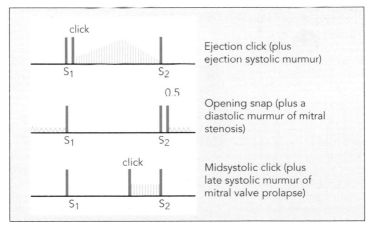

Extra heart sounds.

Other extra heart sounds
Ejection click

This is a high-pitched ringing sound that follows very shortly after the first heart sound. It is a feature of aortic or pulmonary valve stenosis, in which it is probably caused by the sudden opening of the deformed valve.

Opening snap
This is a diastolic sound heard in mitral stenosis and associated with the tensing of the diaphragm formed by the stenosed mitral valve. It is best heard to the left of the sternum.

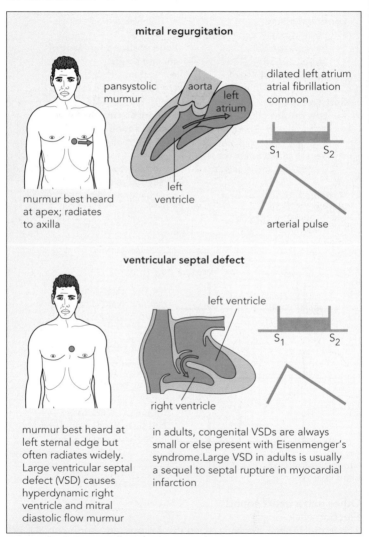

mitral regurgitation

pansystolic murmur

aorta

left atrium

dilated left atrium atrial fibrillation common

left ventricle

S_1 S_2

murmur best heard at apex; radiates to axilla

arterial pulse

ventricular septal defect

left ventricle

S_1 S_2

right ventricle

murmur best heard at left sternal edge but often radiates widely. Large ventricular septal defect (VSD) causes hyperdynamic right ventricle and mitral diastolic flow murmur

in adults, congenital VSDs are always small or else present with Eisenmenger's syndrome. Large VSD in adults is usually a sequel to septal rupture in myocardial infarction

Pansystolic (holosystolic) murmurs: mitral regurgitation (top), ventricular septal defect (lower).

Midsystolic clicks

These are usually associated with mitral valve prolapse and are caused by the tensing of the long and redundant chordae tendineae of these valves. The clicks may or may not be associated with a late systolic murmur.

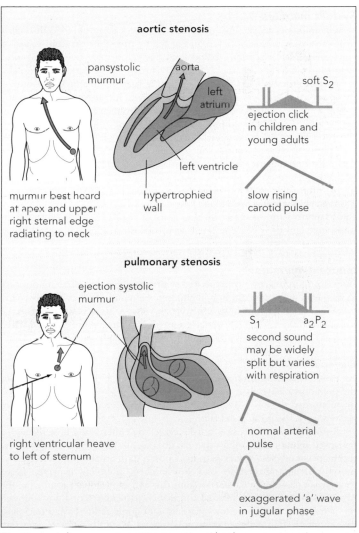

Ejection systolic murmurs: aortic stenosis and pulmonary stenosis.

Murmurs

The important points in analysing a murmur are where it occurs in the cardiac cycle, what it sounds like, where it is best heard, where it radiates to and what happens to manoeuvres like deep breathing.

Systolic murmurs

Systolic murmurs are due to one of three things: leakage of blood through a structure that is normally closed during systole (mitral or tricuspid valves or the interventricular septum), blood flow through a valve normally open in systole but which has become abnormally narrowed (e.g. aortic or pulmonary stenosis) or increased blood flow through a normal valve (a flow murmur).

Murmurs due to leakage of blood through an incompetent mitral or tricuspid valve or a ventricular septal defect are of similar intensity throughout the length of systole. They are called pansystolic or holosystolic. Occasionally, a valve is competent at the start of systole but starts to leak half way through. This is common in patients with mitral valve prolapse. The result is a murmur that starts in mid- or late systole and is called a midsystolic or late systolic murmur, respectively.

Murmurs due to blood being forced through a narrow aortic or pulmonary valve or to increased blood flow through a normal aortic or pulmonary valve tend to start quietly at the beginning of systole, rise to a crescendo in midsystole and then become quiet again towards the end of systole. Such murmurs are called ejection systolic murmurs.

Innocent murmurs

Innocent murmurs are not associated with any major structural abnormality in the heart. They are common in children and young adults. They have the following characteristics: always systolic and always quiet (less than grade 3), usually best heard at the left sternal edge, no associated ventricular hypertrophy, and normal heart sounds, pulses, chest radiograph and ECG.

Diastolic murmurs

An early diastolic murmur is caused by incompetence of either the aortic or the pulmonary valve. It is maximal at the beginning of diastole when aortic or pulmonary pressure is highest and rapidly becomes quieter (decrescendo) as pressure in the great vessel falls.

A mid-diastolic murmur is usually caused by either blood flow through a narrowed mitral or tricuspid valve or, occasionally, to increased blood flow through one of these valves (e.g. in children with atrial septal defect). The murmur of mitral stenosis is a low-pitched, rumbling murmur heard throughout diastole. In patients in sinus rhythm, it gets louder just before the onset of systole as a result of atrial contraction increasing blood flow through the narrowed valve. Sometimes patients with aortic reflux have a mid-diastolic murmur. This is caused by the regurgitant blood from the incompetent aortic valve setting up a vibration of the anterior leaflet of the mitral valve (Austin Flint murmur).

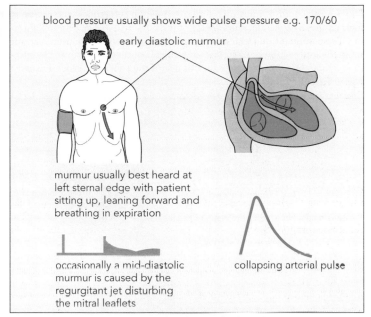

blood pressure usually shows wide pulse pressure e.g. 170/60

early diastolic murmur

murmur usually best heard at
left sternal edge with patient
sitting up, leaning forward and
breathing in expiration

occasionally a mid-diastolic
murmur is caused by the
regurgitant jet disturbing
the mitral leaflets

collapsing arterial pulse

Aortic regurgitation as an example of an early diastolic murmur.

It is sometimes possible to make murmurs easier to hear by putting the patient into special positions. The murmur of mitral stenosis is best heard if the patient is rolled onto his or her left side. The murmur of aortic reflux is sometimes best heard if the patient is made to sit up, lean forward and breathe out fully.

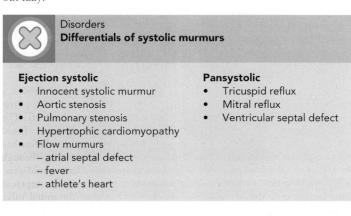

Disorders
Differentials of systolic murmurs

Ejection systolic
- Innocent systolic murmur
- Aortic stenosis
- Pulmonary stenosis
- Hypertrophic cardiomyopathy
- Flow murmurs
  – atrial septal defect
  – fever
  – athlete's heart

Pansystolic
- Tricuspid reflux
- Mitral reflux
- Ventricular septal defect

The behaviour of murmurs during respiration sometimes gives a clue to their nature. Systolic murmurs arising at the pulmonary valve get louder during inspiration and quieter during expiration. Conversely, murmurs arising on the left side of the heart tend to get quieter during inspiration. The murmur of mitral stenosis is often easier to hear if the patient is made to exercise before listening for it.

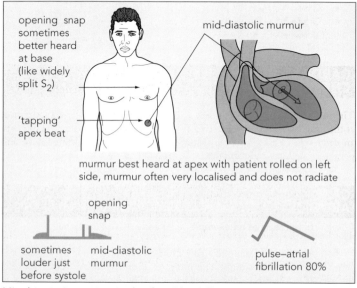

opening snap sometimes better heard at base (like widely split S_2)

'tapping' apex beat

mid-diastolic murmur

murmur best heard at apex with patient rolled on left side, murmur often very localised and does not radiate

opening snap

sometimes louder just before systole

mid-diastolic murmur

pulse–atrial fibrillation 80%

Mitral stenosis as an example of a midsystolic murmur.

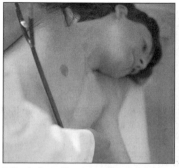

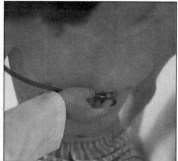

Mitral diastolic murmurs are best heard using the bell, with the patient rolled onto the left side. Aortic diastolic murmurs may be heard more easily if the patient sits up, leans forward and holds his or her breath in expiration.

Summary
Grading the intensity of murmurs

- Grade 1 just audible with a good stethoscope in a quiet room
- Grade 2 quiet but readily audible with a stethoscope
- Grade 3 easily heard with a stethoscope
- Grade 4 a loud, obvious murmur
- Grade 5 very loud, heard not only over the precordium but elsewhere in the body

CARDIOVASCULAR SYSTEM AND CHEST EXAMINATION

The most important feature in cardiac disease is the presence of crepitations at the lung bases. These are crackling sounds during inspiration and they are an early sign of pulmonary oedema. Patients with severe heart failure and peripheral oedema may also develop pleural effusions.

CARDIOVASCULAR SYSTEM AND ABDOMINAL EXAMINATION

The liver will enlarge in response to any rise in right atrial pressure. If the enlargement is rapid, this leads to acute discomfort in the right upper quadrant of the abdomen. In tricuspid reflux, there is a marked hepatic pulsation in time with the regurgitation waves in the jugular venous pulse.

In severe heart failure, the spleen may also become passively enlarged. Enlargement of the spleen is seen in subacute bacterial endocarditis.

Aneurysm of the abdominal aorta is common; the finding on examination is pulsation at about the level of the umbilicus. Use abdominal ultrasound examination to confirm the diagnosis of aortic aneurysm and measure its size.

Enlarged kidneys caused by polycystic disease sometimes present as hypertension. Another cause of hypertension is renal artery stenosis; it is sometimes possible to hear a murmur or bruit to one side or other of the umbilicus.

PERIPHERAL VASCULAR SYSTEM

Assess the skin temperature in the feet and feel the popliteal and dorsalis pedis pulses. Look for varicose veins and for the presence of oedema.

OEDEMA

Heart failure is an important cause of oedema. The oedema of heart failure is largely the result of increased venous pressure, and abnormal capillary permeability may also play a role.

Peripheral oedema is usually a feature of right-sided heart failure or congestive heart failure. It accumulates at the lowest part of the body ('dependent oedema'), namely, the feet and ankles in ambulant patients and the sacrum in patients confined to bed. Severe oedema is frequently accompanied by increased leakage of fluid into the serous cavities and may be accompanied by ascites and pleural effusions. The main differential diagnosis of cardiac oedema is stasis oedema which occurs in elderly or immobile patients. The distinction is made by looking for other signs of cardiac failure.

CLINICAL FEATURES OF SPECIFIC CARDIAC CONDITIONS

HEART FAILURE
Acute heart failure
The most common manifestation of acute heart failure is a low systemic blood pressure. Sometimes intense peripheral vasoconstriction supports a normal or even increased blood pressure. Acute left heart failure is accompanied by pulmonary oedema. The patient becomes extremely breathless, develops a cough and may produce frothy pink-stained sputum. The sign of pulmonary oedema is widespread crepitations or crackling sounds best heard at the base of the lungs. The chest radiograph shows white fluffy shadows in both lungs. With acute right heart failure, for example, as a consequence of acute massive pulmonary embolism, there is no pulmonary oedema but the jugular venous pressure is elevated.

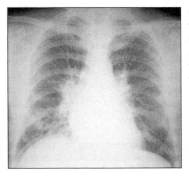

Chest radiograph of acute left heart failure caused by mitral stenosis (Note, left heart failure does not equate with left ventricular failure: the left ventricle in mitral stenosis is fine!)

Chronic heart failure
In chronic left heart failure, there is often a reflex rise in pulmonary vascular resistance, protecting the patient from pulmonary oedema at the cost of precipitating secondary right heart failure. This combination is sometimes called mixed or congestive heart failure.

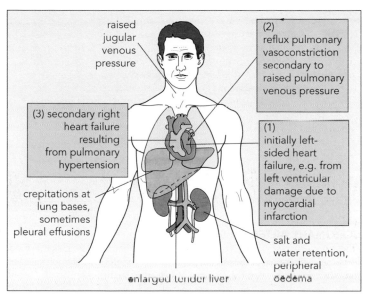

raised jugular venous pressure

(2) reflux pulmonary vasoconstriction secondary to raised pulmonary venous pressure

(3) secondary right heart failure resulting from pulmonary hypertension

(1) initially left-sided heart failure, e.g. from left ventricular damage due to myocardial infarction

crepitations at lung bases, sometimes pleural effusions

salt and water retention, peripheral oedema

enlarged tender liver

Mixed or 'congestive' heart failure starts as left heart failure, but secondary pulmonary vasoconstriction then causes right heart failure.

Summary
Clinical features of acute heart failure

- Acute dyspnoea (pulmonary oedema)
- Hypotension (may be marked by general vasoconstriction)
- Cold clammy skin (peripheral vasoconstriction)
- Anxiety
- Confusion (impaired cerebral blood flow, hypoxaemia)
- Oliguria

Summary
Clinical features of chronic heart failure

- Fatigue on minimal exertion
- Exertional dyspnoea
- Peripheral oedema
- Abdominal discomfort (from hepatic distension)
- Nocturia (reversal of diurnal rhythm)
- Weight loss and cachexia

Risk factors
Coronary artery disease

Inherited
- Familial hyperlipidaemia
- High lipoprotein a (e.g. Indo origin)
- Others[1]

Acquired
- Smoking
- Acquired hyperlipidaemia
- Diabetes
- Hypertension
- Physical inactivity

[1] This includes many common polymorphisms with small (but cumulative) effects and some rare polymorphisms (e.g. pseudoxanthoma elasticum) with large effects.

CORONARY ARTERY DISEASE
Angina

Physical examination of the angina patient is frequently entirely normal. The examiner should be alert for features of hyperlipidaemia.

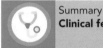

Summary
Clinical features of hyperlipidaemia

Common
- Corneal arcus (nonspecific in patients over 50 years old)
- Xanthelasma (nonspecific in patients over 50 years old)
- Tendon xanthomas (mainly in familial hypercholesterolaemia)

Less common
- Palmar xanthomas
- Eruptive xanthomas
- Ejection systolic murmur (familial hypercholesterolaemia)
- Lipaemia retinalis

Myocardial infarction

The patient may previously have suffered from angina, but frequently this is not the case. The most characteristic symptom of myocardial infarction is chest pain which is similar in distribution to the pain of angina but is usually much more severe and persists even when the patient rests. In a small proportion of patients, myocardial infarction can be relatively painless.

The main risk in the early stages is ventricular fibrillation. Later complications include arrhythmias, cardiac rupture and, occasionally, the development of ventricular septal defect or mitral reflux.

Summary
Clinical features of acute myocardial infarction

Symptoms
- Severe pain
- Pain persists despite rest

Physical signs
- Signs of sympathetic activation (pallor, sweating)
- Narrow pulse pressures
- May be extrasystoles
- May be added (third) heart sound

PERIPHERAL VASCULAR DISEASE

Acute arterial obstruction presents with a cold, white, painful, pulseless limb. The site of obstruction is usually obvious from examining the pulses. Embolism may be the first clue to a cardiac disease such as atrial myxoma.

Chronic arterial insufficiency usually presents as intermittent claudication. The patient is aware of pain either in the leg, the thigh or the buttock which comes on with walking and goes away when stopping to rest. Examination of the leg reveals weak or absent foot, knee and sometimes femoral pulses. There may be a murmur or bruit over the femoral artery. As the disease progresses, pain comes on with progressively less exertion until finally the patient experiences pain at rest. Pain is often worse at night. The skin tends to become discoloured and shiny, and hair is lost from the foot. Infection spreads rapidly. Eventually, gangrene may affect the toes and foot.

DISEASES OF THE PERIPHERAL VEINS
Varicose veins
Varicose veins are excessively dilated superficial leg veins. The two major causes of varicose veins are defective valves in the 'perforating veins' which connect the deep and superficial venous systems in the calf, and defective valves in the upper part of the long saphenous vein where it joins the femoral vein at the thigh.

Varicose veins are always most apparent when the patient is standing and empty when the legs are raised above heart level. By elevating the legs to empty the veins and then watching the veins fill as the leg is lowered, it is often possible to see the sites of incompetent perforating veins and to control them by local finger pressure. If the saphenofemoral junction is incompetent, it may be necessary first to prevent blood flowing back from the femoral vein by tying a tourniquet around the upper thigh.

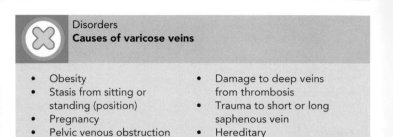

Disorders
Causes of varicose veins

- Obesity
- Stasis from sitting or standing (position)
- Pregnancy
- Pelvic venous obstruction
- Damage to deep veins from thrombosis
- Trauma to short or long saphenous vein
- Hereditary

Chronic venous insufficiency

Failure or inadequacy of the 'muscle pump' mechanism may also lead to chronic oedema of the legs and feet, with or without obvious varicose veins. The oedema is often relatively firm and pits only reluctantly on pressure; it is usually least apparent in the morning and gets worse as the day goes on. The condition is distinguished from heart failure because the jugular venous pressure is normal.

Varicose ulceration and eczema

Chronic venous insufficiency results in a rise in tissue pressure in the skin and subcutaneous tissues which can interfere with adequate nutrient blood flow. This may lead to skin necrosis and ulceration, most commonly at the ankle just above the malleoli. The skin is often dusky and indurated.

Thrombophlebitis

Superficial thrombophlebitis is inflammation and thrombosis of a superficial vein. There is local pain, redness and tenderness over the course of the vein. Septic thrombophlebitis from a drip site infection can lead to septicaemia.

Deep vein thrombosis

Thrombosis of the deep veins in the calf or pelvis usually occurs as a result of a combination of damage to the endothelial lining of the veins, with stasis of the blood within them as a consequence of physical inactivity. In some patients, deep vein thrombosis occurs in the absence of any obvious external

Disorders
Differential diagnosis of deep vein thrombosis

Pain and swelling in the leg may be caused by:
- deep vein thrombosis
- ruptured head of gastrocnemius muscle
- ruptured osteoarthritic cyst (Baker's cyst) of knee joint
- anterior compartment syndrome (skin splints)

cause; it is important that these patients should be investigated for abnormalities of the blood clotting and fibrinolytic systems.

The characteristic clinical features of deep vein thrombosis in the leg are pain, swelling and occasionally redness. The pain is a deep aching pain; sometimes it is absent. There is often dilatation of the superficial veins and a warm skin as a result of blood.

If pain and swelling are below the knee, then it is likely that the thrombosis is in the calf veins. If the swelling and tenderness extend to the thigh or the groin, the thrombosis may involve the femoral or iliac veins.

Acute pulmonary infarction

This is usually the consequence of a pulmonary embolus, a wedge-shaped section of the lung that becomes necrotic. This induces pleural inflammation and the resulting pleurisy causes pain. The presentation is with the relatively sudden onset of pleuritic chest pain. The patient may be moderately breathless. It is important to look for other evidence of deep vein thrombosis both by clinical examination and by phlebography.

Acute massive pulmonary embolism

This is most common in postoperative patients. The patient suddenly becomes extremely short of breath, severely hypotensive and may not be able to sit upright. The jugular veins are markedly distended and the liver may also be enlarged. There may be a third sound best heard to the left of the sternum. Definitive diagnosis is by pulmonary angiography.

Chronic pulmonary hypertension

The clinical features are of chronic pulmonary hypertension. The diagnosis can sometimes be made on the basis of recurrent history of deep vein thrombosis.

INFECTIVE ENDOCARDITIS

Infective endocarditis is an infection of the endocardial lining of the heart.

Acute endocarditis

The result of infection of a normal or abnormal heart with a virulent organism such as *Staphylococcus aureuss* or *Streptococcus pneumoniae*. The infection may cause destruction of valve tissue, abscess formation or the formation of large vegetations. The patient is severely ill with a fever and marked systemic symptoms. The characteristic clinical finding is that heart murmurs develop or change rapidly as the destructive process goes on. There may also be systemic emboli. There may be finger clubbing and splinter haemorrhages but often they do not have time to develop.

Subacute endocarditis

Subacute endocarditis may result either from infection of a diseased heart valve or septal defect with an indolent organism, such as *Streptococcus sanguis*. The illness is much more insidious. Patients present with unexplained fever, tiredness, depressive symptoms or with the consequences of valve destruction or systemic embolisation. There is nearly always a heart murmur: the combination of fever and a heart murmur should always lead to suspicion of endocarditis. The murmurs may change over a time course of days or weeks rather than hours. Finger clubbing and splinter haemorrhages are common. There may be anaemia and there is often splenomegaly. There may be localised subconjunctival haemorrhages, tender swellings (Osler's nodes) in the finger pulps and haemorrhagic spots (Roth spots) in the retina. All are features of a systemic vasculitis.

MYOCARDITIS

Myocarditis is an inflammatory infection of heart muscle, usually the result of a virus infection. Clinically, this may present with heart failure or an arrhythmia. There may be cardiac dilatation, a third heart sound or a systolic murmur from 'functional' mitral incompetence resulting from dilatation of the ventricle.

CARDIOMYOPATHY

Cardiomyopathy is a general term meaning 'heart muscle disease'.

Hypertrophic cardiomyopathy

Hypertrophic cardiomyopathy is characterised by excessive cardiac muscle hypertrophy in the absence of a stimulus such as hypertension. The hypertrophy specifically affects the interventricular septum, which bulges into the left ventricular outflow tract and causes obstruction to blood flow.

Dilated cardiomyopathy

This is characterised by a global impairment of left ventricular function, leading to progressive dilatation of the ventricles. The basic cause is unknown but similar patterns can be reproduced in association with excessive alcohol intake or systemic diseases (e.g. sarcoidois). There is a displaced apex beat, a gallop rhythm and possibly secondary mitral or tricuspid regurgitation.

Restrictive cardiomyopathy

The clinical presentation mimics constrictive pericarditis.

ACUTE RHEUMATIC FEVER

Clinically, acute rheumatic fever presents in children or young adults either with an acute, migratory (i.e. flitting from joint to joint) polyarthritis or with chorea.

Cardiac involvement is usually signalled by a pansystolic murmur of mitral regurgitation or a soft mid-diastolic murmur that resembles that of mitral stenosis (called a Carey Coombs murmur) and caused by oedema of the mitral valve cusps and by small platelet vegetations. There is commonly a skin rash. Rheumatic nodules consist of firm subcutaneous nodules on the extensor surfaces of knees and elbows.

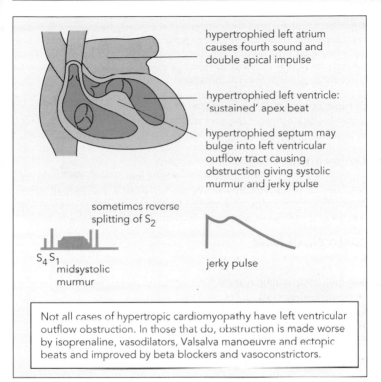

hypertrophied left atrium causes fourth sound and double apical impulse

hypertrophied left ventricle: 'sustained' apex beat

hypertrophied septum may bulge into left ventricular outflow tract causing obstruction giving systolic murmur and jerky pulse

sometimes reverse splitting of S_2

$S_4 S_1$
midsystolic murmur

jerky pulse

Not all cases of hypertropic cardiomyopathy have left ventricular outflow obstruction. In those that do, obstruction is made worse by isoprenaline, vasodilators, Valsalva manoeuvre and ectopic beats and improved by beta blockers and vasoconstrictors.

Findings in hypertrophic cardiomyopathy.

PERICARDIAL DISEASE
Acute pericarditis

The most characteristic physical finding is the pericardial rub. Pericardial rubs are often best heard if the patient is made to sit up, lean forward and breathe out fully. It is characteristic of a pericardial rub in that it comes and goes over a period of a few hours. Patients with acute pericarditis are often pyrexic and may feel systemically unwell.

Pericardial effusion

A large amount of fluid or the very rapid accumulation of fluid causes compression of the heart, particularly the right ventricle, and can cause a substantial reduction in cardiac output. This is cardiac tamponade. The patient is often very ill, hypotensive and peripherally constricted. There may be pulsus paradoxus: a variation in pulse volume with respiration. The jugular venous pressure is very high.

If fluid accumulates slowly in the pericardium over days or weeks, then it is often accommodated by stretching of the pericardium rather than cardiac tamponade. It presents as chronic predominantly right-sided cardiac failure, often with very marked peripheral oedema and perhaps ascites. There may or may not be a pericardial rub. The jugular venous pressure is usually markedly elevated. There may be a paradoxical pulse

Chronic constrictive pericarditis

Chronic inflammation of the pericardium may lead to a thickened fibrotic pericardial membrane which constricts and compresses the heart. The most common cause of this is chronic tuberculous pericarditis but it may also follow acute viral pericarditis or cardiac surgery.

There tends to be predominantly right-sided heart failure often with massive oedema. The jugular venous pressure is elevated and often has a characteristic pulse wave-form, with a very rapid dip in the pulse as the tricuspid valve opens followed by an equally abrupt termination as filling of the ventricle is curtailed.

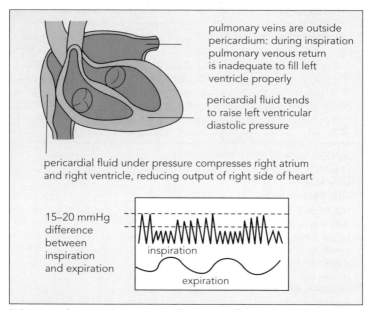

pulmonary veins are outside pericardium: during inspiration pulmonary venous return is inadequate to fill left ventricle properly

pericardial fluid tends to raise left ventricular diastolic pressure

pericardial fluid under pressure compresses right atrium and right ventricle, reducing output of right side of heart

15–20 mmHg difference between inspiration and expiration

inspiration

expiration

Pulses paradoxus or the apparent diminuition of the pulse on inspiration is a feature of pericardial tamponade.

Examination of elderly people
Cardiovascular examination

No one is too old or too ill for a proper cardiovascular examination and diagnosis. Neither the approach or the technique of cardiovascular examination for elderly people differs significantly from that adopted for younger patients. Older patients tend to be less mobile and techniques such as treadmill exercise testing may be impracticable but alternatives such as pharmacological stress testing are available. The main differences lie in the increased prevalence of cardiovascular pathology, the frequency of multisystem disease and in the interpretation of particular findings.

Hypertension, ischaemic heart disease and peripheral vascular disease are all more common in elderly people. Ischaemic heart disease is often asymptomatic because patients do not exercise enough to give themselves angina. 'Silent' myocardial infarction is also more frequent in elderly people. Heart failure is more prevalent among older people but the most common cause of ankle oedema in the elderly is not heart failure but venous insufficiency and stasis. Heart failure should never be diagnosed on the basis of ankle swelling alone. Valvular heart disease, particularly calcific aortic stenosis, is common. Aortic stenosis is an important diagnosis to make, because aortic valve replacement can be carried out safely and effectively even in elderly patients. Neither blood pressure nor pulse waves are reliable guides to the severity of aortic stenosis in elderly patients and proper evaluation, e.g. by ECG, is important before a murmur is written off as 'innocent'. Cardiac arrhythmias, particularly ventricular or atrial extrasystoles, or short runs of self-terminating atrial fibrillation, are common in elderly people and seldom associated with symptoms. They do not need detailed investigation unless they are obviously relevant to the patient's history.

One complaint that is particulary frequent in elderly patients is dizziness or transient loss of consciousness. Possible causes include postural hypotension which may be spontaneous or drug induced, vertebrobasilar insufficiency as a result of cervical spondylosis or a cardiac arrhythmia, most often a slow (brady) rather than a fast (tachy) arrhythmia, which is most commonly detected by Holter monitoring.

Remember that elderly patients often have multiple pathology and may be taking a variety of medications. Some of these may themselves cause cardiovascular problems, e.g. nonsteroidal anti-inflammatory drugs can cause fluid retention and put up blood pressure. Decisions to offer specific treatments to elderly patients depend on weighing up the potential advantages against disadvantages in terms of discomfort, risk and cost. Without a proper diagnosis, however, rational decisions cannot be made.

Disorders
Causes of pericardial effusion

Infection
- Viral pericarditis
- Bacterial pericarditis (streptococcus)
- Tuberculosis pericarditis

Myocardial infarction
- Peri-infarct pericarditis
- Cardiac rupture
- Dressler's syndrome

Malignant pericarditis
- Secondary (common) or primary (rare) tumours
- Leukaemia

Auto-allergic
- Acute rheumatic fever
- Rheumatoid arthritis

Other
- Myxoedema
- Trauma (stab wounds)
- After cardiac surgery

7. The Abdomen

Diseases of the abdominal organs may already be apparent from the general examination when you may have noticed jaundice. You may also have been aware of abnormal weight loss, signs of malnutrition or anaemia.

SYMPTOMS OF ABDOMINAL DISORDERS

GASTROINTESTINAL DISEASES
Dysphagia

Determine whether the dysphagia developed suddenly or gradually over weeks or months whether the symptom is constant or intermittent and whether the dysphagia occurs with both solids and liquids. Associated symptoms such as weight loss and pain or cough with swallowing may help you construct a differential diagnosis.

Dysphagia caused by a carcinoma usually progresses rapidly over 6–10 weeks and is worse for solids than liquids. Profound weight loss results from reduced food intake and the wasting effect of the cancer.

✗ Disorders
Causes of dysphagia

- Benign oesophageal stricture
- Carcinoma of the oesophagus
- Achalasia of the cardia or motility disorders
- Systemic sclerosis
- Old age (presbyoesophagus)
- Bulbar and pseudobulbar palsy

? Questions to ask
Dysphagia

- At what level does food stick?
- Has the symptom developed over weeks, months or longer?
- Is the dysphagia intermittent or progressive?
- Are both food and drink equally difficult to swallow?
- Is there a history of reflux symptoms?

Patients with a benign 'peptic' stricture often have a long history of heart-burn, a slower rate of progression and less marked weight loss. Achalasia of the cardia may be particularly difficult to distinguish, although some patients report that the symptom fluctuates in intensity and that the dysphagia is equal for liquids and solids. When dysphagia is caused by pseudobulbar palsy or bulbar palsy it is accompanied by coughing and spluttering.

Heartburn

The pain is a scalding or burning sensation that wells up behind the sternum and radiates towards the throat. An acid or bitter taste may develop in the mouth and reflex salivation may cause it to fill with saliva (water brash). A common cause of heartburn is a hiatus hernia. The heartburn is often provoked by postures which raise intra-abdominal pressure such as stooping, bending or lying down. It is a common symptom in the later months of pregnancy.

Pain on swallowing (odynophagia)

The symptom suggests intense spasm of the oesophagus; it may be caused by an intrinsic motor disorder causing intense and uncoordinated contraction ('nutcracker' oesophagus).

Loss of appetite (anorexia)

A nonspecific symptom that commonly accompanies both acute and chronic ill health. Prolonged or unexplained anorexia, when accompanied by weight loss, should alert you to a serious underlying disease. Anorexia may be a prominent feature of digestive diseases, failure of the major organs (kidneys, liver, heart and lungs) and generalised debilitating illnesses (e.g. cancer, tuberculosis).

Anorexia nervosa results in marked weight loss, malnutrition and cessa-tion of menstruation (amenorrhoea). Suspect anorexia nervosa in teenagers and young adults who present with depression, vomiting or purgative abuse.

Weight loss

Weight loss is an important but rather unspecific symptom of gastrointestinal and other diseases. Weight loss may be caused by inappropriate wastage of calories due to steatorrhoea, thyrotoxicosis or diabetes mellitus.

Dyspepsia and indigestion

Most often these terms apply to a sensation of pain, discomfort or fullness in the epigastrium, frequently accompanied by belching, nausea or heartburn. Determine the character and timing, the aggravating and relieving factors and the associated symptoms.

Nausea

Nausea describes the sensation experienced before vomiting, although it often occurs without vomiting. It may be relieved by vomiting.

Questions to ask
Weight loss

- Is your appetite normal, increased or decreased?
- Over what timespan has the weight been lost?
- Do you enjoy your meals?
- Describe your usual breakfast, lunch and supper.
- Is the weight loss associated with nausea, vomiting or abdominal pain?
- Are your motions normal in colour and consistency?
- Has there been a fever?
- Do you pass excessive volumes of urine?
- Have you noticed a recent change in weather tolerance?

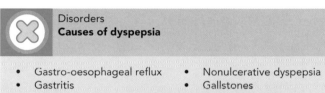

Disorders
Causes of dyspepsia

- Gastro-oesophageal reflux
- Gastritis
- Peptic ulcer disease
- Nonulcerative dyspepsia
- Gallstones
- Pancreatitis

Vomiting and haematemesis

Vomiting may occur in diseases of the gastrointestinal and biliary tracts, as well as in a variety of systemic and metabolic disorders. It may also be the presenting symptom of psychological disorders such as anorexia nervosa and bulimia. Suspect an iatrogenic cause in patients taking digoxin or morphine. The presence of undigested food and a lack of bile suggest pyloric obstruction. Early morning nausea and vomiting are characteristic of early pregnancy and alcoholism.

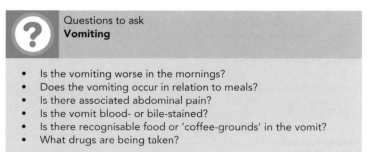

Questions to ask
Vomiting

- Is the vomiting worse in the mornings?
- Does the vomiting occur in relation to meals?
- Is there associated abdominal pain?
- Is the vomit blood- or bile-stained?
- Is there recognisable food or 'coffee-grounds' in the vomit?
- What drugs are being taken?

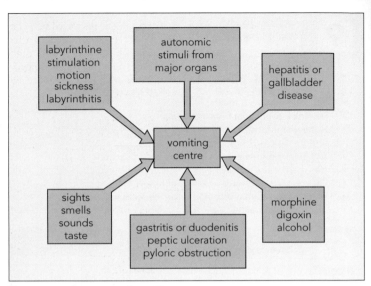

The causes of nausea and vomiting.

Vomiting blood (haematemesis) indicates bleeding from the oesophagus, stomach or duodenum. If the bleeding is preceded by repeated bouts of retching or vomiting, consider a Mallory–Weiss tear. Enquire about ingestion of alcohol or other gastric irritants (e.g. aspirin).

Disorders
Causes of gastrointestinal bleeding

Cause	Frequency
Gastric ulcer	30
Duodenal ulcer	21
Gastritis or erosions	9
Oesophagitis or oesophageal ulcer	8
Duodenitis	4
Varices	3
Tumours	2
Mallory–Weiss tear	1
Others	22

Abdominal pain

When taking a history of abdominal pain, aim to distinguish between visceral, parietal and referred pain.

Visceral pain is often described as a 'dull ache' that is perceived near the midline, irrespective of the location of the organ. The pain can usually be localised to the epigastric, periumbilical or suprapubic areas depending on whether the affected organ is derived from the embryological foregut, midgut or hindgut. Visceral pain may also radiate. It is commonly accompanied by nonspecific, 'visceral' symptoms (e.g. anorexia, nausea, pallor, sweating).

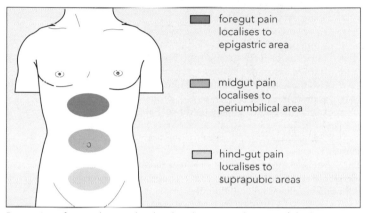

foregut pain localises to epigastric area

midgut pain localises to periumbilical area

hind-gut pain localises to suprapubic areas

Perception of visceral pain is localised to the epigastric, periumbilical or suprapubic region according to the embryological origin of the diseased organ.

Colic signifies obstruction of a hollow, muscular organ such as the intestine, gallbladder, bile duct or ureter. When the smaller organs such as the gallbladder, bile duct or ureters are acutely obstructed by a stone, the cyclical nature of colic soon gives way to a continuous visceral pain caused by the inflammatory effect of the impacted stone or secondary infection. Movement does not aggravate visceral pain.

Pain arising from the parietal peritoneum is well localised to the area immediately overlying the area of inflammation or irritation. Parietal pain is aggravated by stretching or moving the peritoneal membrane; the patient lies as still as possible. Palpation of the area is extremely painful, with the overlying muscles contracting to protect the peritoneum (guarding). When the pressure of the examining hand is suddenly released the pain is further aggravated and the patient winces ('rebound tenderness').

Abdominal pain may progress from a visceral sensation to a parietal pain. Acute appendicitis provides an excellent example of this transition.

Mesenteric angina

When the mesenteric arteries are stenosed the blood supply to the bowel may be impaired. The pain usually becomes apparent only on eating, and causes anorexia, which, together with damage to the bowel mucosa, results in weight loss.

Questions to ask
Abdominal pain

- What is the position and character of the pain, and to where does it radiate?
- Has the pain been present for hours, days, weeks, months or years?
- Is the pain constant or intermittent?
- Have you noticed specific aggravating or relieving factors?
- Is the pain affected by eating or defecation?
- Does the pain awake you from sleep?
- Is there associated nausea or vomiting?
- Has there been associated weight loss?
- Is there a history of ulcerogenic drugs?
- Has there been a change in bowel habit?

Wind

Excessive belching (flatulence) or the passage of wind through the anus (flatus) are common symptoms. These symptoms are unspecific and occur in both functional and organic disorders of the gastrointestinal tract.

Change in bowel habit
Constipation

Constipation is characterised by straining and the infrequent passage of small, hard stools. Constipated patients often complain that they are left with a sense of incomplete evacuation (tenesmus). A history of laxative use may be a helpful guide to the severity of the condition.

When constipation has troubled a patient for years or even decades, the cause is likely to be functional rather than obstructive.

When constipation presents as a recent change, and especially if it is associated with colic, consider an organic cause such as malignancy or stricture formation. Enquire about constipating drugs and about rectal bleeding.

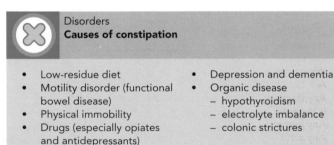

Disorders
Causes of constipation

- Low-residue diet
- Motility disorder (functional bowel disease)
- Physical immobility
- Drugs (especially opiates and antidepressants)
- Depression and dementia
- Organic disease
  - hypothyroidism
  - electrolyte imbalance
  - colonic strictures

Constipation caused by chronic partial obstruction may be punctuated by periods of loose or watery stool. This 'spurious diarrhoea' occurs in elderly patients with faecal impaction and also when colon cancer causes a partial obstruction.

Questions to ask
Constipation

- What is the normal stool frequency?
- Do you strain at stool?
- How long have you been constipated?
- Is there associated abdominal pain, distension, nausea or vomiting?
- Are the stools large or small and pellet shaped?
- Have you noticed intercurrent diarrhoea (spurious diarrhoea)?
- Are any constipating drugs, such as codeine or other opiates, being used?

Diarrhoea

Diarrhoea implies increased stool volume and frequency and a change in consistency from formed to semi-formed, semi-liquid or liquid. Always enquire about the presence of blood and mucus.

Enquire about colour; in fat malabsorption, the stool is pale, malodorous, poorly formed and difficult to flush. Blood and mucus mixed in the stool suggest an infective colitis or inflammatory bowel disease. Consider laxative abuse and recent broad-spectrum antibiotic treatment. Thyrotoxicosis may present with increased stool frequency.

Questions to ask
Diarrhoea

- What is the normal stool frequency?
- How many stools daily?
- How long have you had diarrhoea?
- Are you awoken from sleep to open the bowels?
- What is the colour and consistency of stools?
- Are blood and mucus present?
- Any travel abroad or contact with diarrhoea?
- Is there associated nausea, vomiting, weight loss or pain?
- Any purgative abuse?
- Any antibiotics?

Rectal bleeding

Rectal bleeding is a symptom common to several disorders. Colon cancer and polyps often present with intermittent rectal bleeding, whereas patients with inflammatory bowel disease pass blood, often mixed with mucus, with most stools. Microscopic blood loss (occult bleeding) usually presents with symptoms of anaemia. Haemorrhoids are common, so always consider other causes of bleeding in patients aged 40 and over.

Black stools with the colour and consistency of tar (melena) usually indicate bleeding from the oesophagus, stomach or duodenum. Treatment with iron and certain drugs (e.g. bismuth) also blackens the stool and this cause must be distinguished from melena.

Disorders
Causes of steatorrhoea

- Chronic pancreatitis
- Small bowel bacterial overgrowth
- Gluten enteropathy
- Blind loops
- Short bowel syndrome

Questions to ask
Gastrointestinal bleeding

- Is there a past history of abdominal pain or other gastrointestinal symptoms?
- Is there a history of chronic alcoholism or excessive intake?
- Is there a past history of haematemesis, melena or anaemia?
- Are any nonsteroidals, steroids or proprietary medicines being taken?
- Was the bleeding preceded by intense retching?
- Has there been ingestion of iron or bismuth that stains the stools?

LIVER DISEASE

Liver cell damage and obstruction of the bile duct both have numerous clinical consequences, the most striking of which are jaundice, pale stools and darkening of the urine.

Liver cell damage

Symptoms of liver damage are not very specific and include malaise, fatigue, anorexia and nausea. Viral hepatitis is preceded by prodromes such as fatigue, nausea and a profound distaste for alcohol and cigarettes. Before the onset of jaundice the patient may notice darkening of the urine and lightening of stool colour.

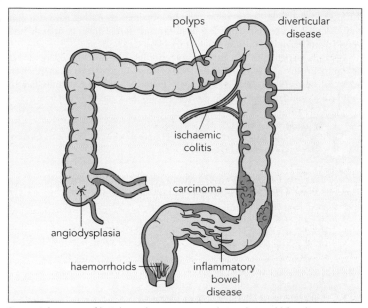

Potential causes of bright red or maroon-coloured rectal bleeding.

Enquire about the principal causes of liver damage. Calculate the number of units (or grams) of alcohol consumed in a week. Ask about foreign travel, intravenous drug abuse or exposure to blood products, and establish the patient's sexual orientation. Enquire about drugs that may cause liver damage and ask about a family history of liver disease.

The patient may notice increasing girth and weight gain caused by the accumulation of ascites. If encephalopathy occurs, the sleep pattern may be reversed and the patient may undergo a change in personality.

BILIARY OBSTRUCTION

The principal symptom is itching (pruritus) and this may occur long before the patient becomes jaundiced. Severe epigastric and right hypochondrial pain accompanied by fever and jaundice suggests impaction of a gallstone in the common bile duct, whereas 'painless' jaundice suggests either a more chronic obstruction of the common bile duct (e.g. cancer of either the bile duct or head of the pancreas) or damage to the intrahepatic biliary tree (e.g. primary biliary cirrhosis, sclerosing cholangitis, drugs). Impaired bile flow into the duodenum causes fat malabsorption and steatorrhoea.

PANCREATIC DISEASE

Acute pancreatitis presents with upper abdominal pain that is most prominent in the epigastrium and left upper quadrant. The pain may radiate through to the back; some relief may be obtained by sitting forward. Ask about alcohol intake and drugs (e.g. azathioprine, furosemide, corticoids) and consider underlying gallstones.

Chronic pancreatitis is often characterised by persistent, severe upper abdominal pain which may radiate to the back. Loss of exocrine function leads to steatorrhoea and weight loss. Diabetes is a late manifestation. Progressive fibrosis may occlude the lower bile duct causing jaundice.

> **?** Questions to ask
> **Jaundice**
>
> - Have you travelled to areas where hepatitis A is endemic?
> - Is there a history of alcohol or intravenous drug abuse?
> - Have you ever had a blood transfusion?
> - Have you had contact with jaundiced patients?
> - Have you experienced skin itching?
> - What medication has been used recently?
> - Have you had occupational contact with hepatotoxins?
> - Is there pain and weight loss?
> - What colour are the stools and urine?
> - Is there a family history of liver disease?

KIDNEY AND BLADDER DISEASE
Frequency and urgency
Frequency refers to the desire to pass urine more often than normal. Urgency may accompany frequency (i.e. a strong urge to urinate even though only small amounts of urine are present in the bladder).

Nocturia
This may occur in patients with daytime frequency or individuals producing excessive quantities of urine (polyuria). Incomplete bladder voiding caused by prostatism often presents with nocturia.

Incontinence
If the symptom is provoked by increased intra–abdominal pressure (coughing, sneezing or laughing), it is referred to as 'stress incontinence'. Diseases causing excessive bladder filling (e.g. bladder outlet obstruction or damage to the nervous supply of the bladder) may cause 'overflow incontinence'.

Hesitancy
A delay between attempting to initiate urination and the actual flow of urine. It is a characteristic sign of bladder outlet obstruction (e.g. as a result of prostatic hypertrophy).

Disorders
Jaundice

Prehepatic or unconjugated hyperbilirubinaemia
- Haemolytic anaemias
- Gilbert's syndrome

Hepatocellular disease
- Viral hepatitis (types A, B, C, D and E)
- Alcoholic hepatitis
- Autoimmune hepatitis (lupoid)
- Drug hepatitis (halothane, paracetamol)
- Decompensated cirrhosis

Intrahepatic cholestasis
- Drugs (phenothiazines)
- Primary biliary cirrhosis
- Primary sclerosing cholangitis

Extrahepatic cholestasis
- Bile duct stricture (benign and malignant)
- Common duct stone
- Cancer of the head of the pancreas

Oliguria and anuria
The term oliguria is used if less than 500 ml of urine is passed over 24 hours.

Pain
Infection of the kidneys (pyelonephritis) causes pain and tenderness in the renal angles, usually associated with fever, anorexia and nausea. Obstruction of the ureters by stones may cause intense pain in the renal angle. Renal 'colic' often causes the patient to double-up or roll around. Bladder pain is of moderate severity, localised to the suprapubic region and associated with urgency and frequency.

Dysuria
A stinging or burning sensation that occurs when passing urine. The most common cause of dysuria is cystitis.

Haematuria
Blood in urine may be obvious, associated with a cloudy colour or only apparent on chemical testing (microscopic haematuria).

Summary
Some renal symptoms and their causes

Frequency
- Irritable bladder
    - infection, inflammation, chemical
    - irritation
- Reduced compliance
    - fibrosis, tumour infiltration
- Bladder outlet obstruction
    - in prostatism, detrusor failure may limit the volume voided

Polyuria
- Ingestion of large volumes of water, beverages or alcohol
- Chronic renal failure (loss of concentrating power)
- Diabetes mellitus (osmotic effect of glucose in urine)
- Diabetes insipidus (caused by a lack of antidiuretic hormone (ADH) or tubules insensitive to circulating ADH)
- Diuretic treatment

Dysuria
- Bacterial infection of the bladder (cystitis)
- Inflammation of the urethra (urethritis)
- Infection or inflammation of the prostate (prostatitis)

Incontinence
- Sphincter damage or weakness after childbirth
- Sphincter weakness in old age
- Prostate cancer
- Benign prostatic hypertrophy
- Spinal cord disease, paraplegia

Oliguria or anuria
- Hypovolaemia (dehydration or shock)
- Acute renal failure caused by acute glomerulonephritis
- Bilateral ureteric obstruction (retroperitoneal fibrosis)
- Detrusor muscle failure (bladder outlet obstruction or neurological disease)

EXAMINATION OF THE ABDOMEN

The abdominal examination depends largely on the palpation and percussion of organs that normally lie out of reach of the examining hands.

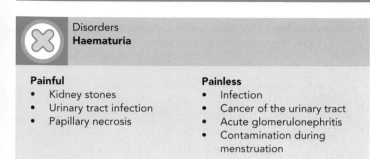

Disorders
Haematuria

Painful
- Kidney stones
- Urinary tract infection
- Papillary necrosis

Painless
- Infection
- Cancer of the urinary tract
- Acute glomerulonephritis
- Contamination during menstruation

A full abdominal examination also includes examination of the lower half of the chest.

For descriptive purposes, the anterior abdominal wall may be divided into four quadrants. The abdomen may also be divided into nine segments resembling a 'noughts and crosses' matrix.

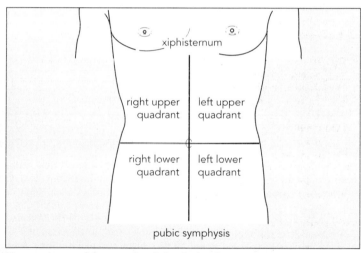

xiphisternum

| right upper quadrant | left upper quadrant |
| right lower quadrant | left lower quadrant |

pubic symphysis

The quadrants of the anterior abdominal wall.

INSPECTION OF THE ABDOMEN
Contours

The normal abdomen is concave and symmetrical. In thin individuals you may notice the pulsation of the abdominal aorta in the midline above the umbilicus.

Fluid gravitates towards the flanks causing the loins to bulge, and the umbilicus, which is normally inverted, may become everted.

The periodic rippling movement of bowel peristalsis may be observed in intestinal obstruction, especially in thin individuals.

Direct and indirect inguinal herniae may also become prominent when intra-abdominal pressure is raised by coughing.

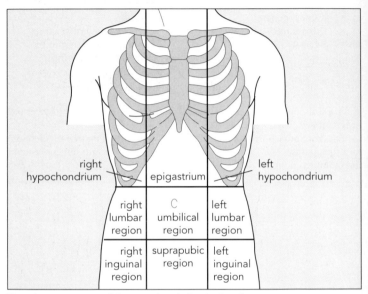

The nine segments of the anterior abdominal wall.

Skin

After childbirth many women are left with tell-tale stretch lines (striae gravidarum). In Cushing's syndrome, purplish striae appear on the abdominal wall. In acute haemorrhagic pancreatitis, there may be a bluish discoloration of either the flanks (Grey Turner's sign) or the periumbilical area (Cullen's sign) which results from seepage of bloodstained ascitic fluid along the fascial planes.

Veins are rarely prominent in health. If visible, map the direction of flow by emptying the vein. The direction of flow helps distinguish normal from abnormal flow patterns.

PALPATION OF THE ABDOMEN

Although the intra-abdominal organs are normally impalpable, in diseased states palpation and percussion provide substantial clinical information. If the abdominal wall muscles are tense, ask the patient to bend the knees and to flex the hips. This helps to relax the abdomen.

A single-handed technique may be used but you may prefer to use both hands, the upper hand applying pressure, while the lower hand concentrates on feeling.

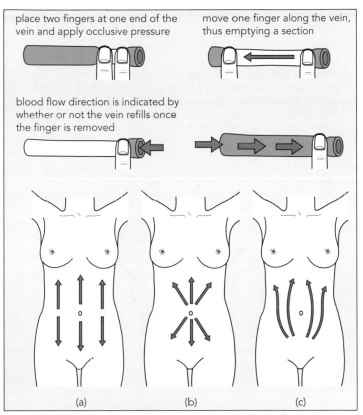

place two fingers at one end of the vein and apply occlusive pressure

move one finger along the vein, thus emptying a section

blood flow direction is indicated by whether or not the vein refills once the finger is removed

(a)   (b)   (c)

Determining the direction of blood flow in abdominal veins. (a) Normal blood flow pattern and those characteristic of (b) portal hypertension and (c) obstruction of the inferior vena cava.

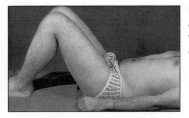

Palpation of the abdomen may be aided if the patient is asked to flex the hips. This helps to relax the anterior abdominal walls.

Light palpation

Ask the patient to localise any areas of pain or tenderness. Begin the examination in the segment furthest from the discomfort.

In peritonitis, the patient flinches on even the lightest palpation and there is reflex rigidity, guarding and rebound tenderness.

Deep palpation

In thin individuals, the descending and sigmoid colon may be felt as an elongated tubular structure in the left loin and lower quadrant. The colon has a putty-like texture and the 'mass' also becomes less obvious after the passage of stool. The abdominal aorta may be felt as a discrete pulsatile structure in the midline, above the umbilicus. A large pulsatile structure in the midline above the umbilicus indicates an aortic aneurysm or a transmitted impulse to a mass overlying the aorta. These can usually be distinguished using the index finger of either hand to sense whether the movement is pulsatile or transmitted.

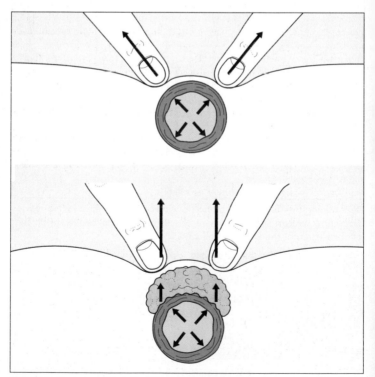

Palpating the aorta. The direction of the pulsation indicates whether it arises directly from the aorta (above) or is transmitted by a mass overlying the tissues (below).

Palpation of the organs
Palpating the liver

Examine the liver with the surface anatomy in mind. Examine from the patient's right and use either the fingertips or the radial side of the index finger at a point midway between the costal margin and iliac crests, lateral to the rectus muscle. Press the fingertips inwards and upwards while the patient takes a deep inspiration; feel for the liver edge slipping under them as the organ descends. If no edge is felt repeat the manoeuvre in a stepwise fashion, each time moving the starting position a little closer to the costal margin. In patients of thin or medium build a normal liver edge may be palpable just below the right costal margin at the height of inspiration.

It is useful to percuss for the lower liver edge. Percuss from the point where you started palpating for the liver. This point normally overlies bowel and should sound resonant. Repeat the percussion in a stepwise manner, each time moving the finger closer to the costal margin until the note becomes duller.

Find the position of the upper margin of the liver so that you can assess the liver span. The upper margin can be located by noting the change in percussion note from the resonance of the lungs to the dullness of the liver. In women this should measure 8–10 cm and in men, 10–12 cm.

In patients who have hyperinflated lungs (e.g. emphysema), the liver is pushed down so that the edge may be easily palpable below the costal margin. Percussion reveals that the upper border of the liver is depressed and that the liver span is within normal limits.

The right lobe of the liver may be abnormally shaped. This anatomical variant is known as a Reidel's lobe.

If the liver is enlarged, trace the shape of the liver edge and decide whether it is smooth or irregular, whether the consistency is soft, firm or hard and whether or not the organ is tender. The presence of a palpable spleen suggests cirrhosis with portal hypertension.

The lower margin of the liver may not be palpable because of fibrosis or atrophy of the organ. This should be suspected if the liver edge is not palpable and if, on percussion, the dullness of the lower liver margin is detected well above the costal margin.

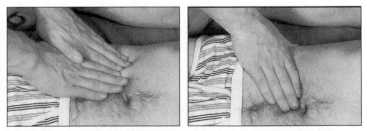

Liver palpation. A two-handed (left) and single-handed (right) technique using the radial surface of the index finger(s) to feel for the lower liver edge as it descends during inspiration.

Disorders
Causes of hepatomegaly

- Macronodular cirrhosis
- Neoplastic disease (primary and secondary cancer, myeloproliferative disorders)
- Infections (viral hepatitis, tuberculosis, hydatid disease)
- Infiltrations (iron, fat, amyloid, Gaucher's disease)
- Congestive heart failure

General signs of liver disease

The physical sign characteristic of hepatic encephalopathy is a 'flapping tremor'. Ask the patient to stretch out both arms and hyperextend the wrists with the fingers held separated. A coarse, involuntary flap occurs at the wrist and metacarpophalangeal joints.

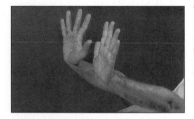

To elicit a flapping tremor in hepatic encephalopathy, ask the patient to outstretch the arms with the hands extended at the wrist and metacarpophalangeal joints. This is held for 20 seconds.

Disorders
Causes of hepatic encephalopathy

- Protein load (acute bleed, dietary binge)
- Diuretics and electrolyte abnormalities
- Development of hepatocellular cancer
- Toxins or drugs (alcohol binge, sedatives, opiates)
- Infection

Palpating the gallbladder

Imagine the position of the fundus under the point where the rectus abdominis muscle intersects the costal margin. This surface marking coincides with the tip of the right ninth rib.

Using gentle but firm pressure palpate the gallbladder area by pointing the tips of the fingers towards the organ while the patient inspires deeply. When the gallbladder is inflamed the patient experiences intense pain, winces and interrupts the breath (Murphy's sign).

Summary
Signs of liver disease

General examination
- Nutritional status
- Pallor (blood loss)
- Jaundice
- Breath fetor of liver failure
- Xanthelasmata (chronic cholestasis)
- Parotid swelling (alcohol misuse)
- Bruising (clotting diathesis)
- Spider naevi
- Female distribution of body hair

Mental state
- Wernicke's or Korsakoff's psychosis
- Flapping tremor of hepatic encephalopathy
- Inability to copy a five-pointed star

Hands
- Leukonychia (hypoproteinaemia)
- Liver flap
- Palmar erythema
- Dupuytren's contracture
- Mild finger clubbing

Chest
- Gynaecomastia
- Right-sided pleural effusion

Abdomen
- Dilated veins
- Liver or spleen enlargement
- Ascites
- Testicular atrophy

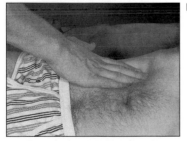

Palpating the gallbladder.

The gallbladder only becomes palpable when obstructed and distended with bile. The distended organ is contiguous with the lower border of the liver and moves with respiration.

Palpating the spleen

The spleen enlarges from under the left costal margin towards the right iliac fossa in a downward and medial direction.

The general technique is similar to that described for the liver. Using a

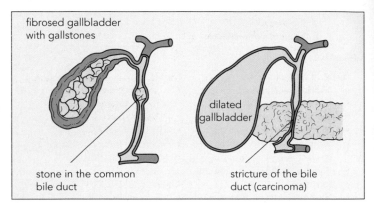

fibrosed gallbladder
with gallstones

dilated
gallbladder

stone in the common
bile duct

stricture of the bile
duct (carcinoma)

If jaundice is caused by impaction of a gallstone in the bile duct, the fibrosed, stone-filled gallbladder does not dilate. However, if jaundice is caused by a bile duct stricture the healthy gallbladder dilates and can be palpated as a soft mass arising from behind the ninth right rib anteriorly.

⊗ Disorders
Causes of portal hypertension

Presinusoidal
- Portal vein block
- Schistosomiasis
- Cystic fibrosis

Sinusoidal and postsinusoidal
- Cirrhosis
- Veno-occlusive disease
- Hepatic vein block (Budd–Chiari syndrome)

moderate amount of pressure, ask the patient to breathe in deeply. The notched leading edge of an enlarged spleen can be felt. If the spleen is impalpable at the starting point of the examination, move the fingertips progressively closer to the left lower rib cage.

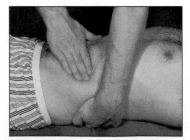

When palpating the spleen use your left hand to support the ribcage posteriorly, while the fingertips of your right hand explore the leading edge of the organ.

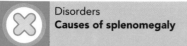

Disorders
Causes of splenomegaly

- Portal hypertension
- Infections (malaria, subacute bacterial endocarditis, tuberculosis, typhoid)
- Chronic lymphatic leukaemia
- Chronic myeloid leukaemia
- Myelofibrosis
- Gaucher's disease
- Haemolytic anaemia

For splenic dullness percuss the ninth intercostal space anterior to the anterior axillary line (Traub's space). This space is normally tympanitic but as the solid spleen enlarges this area becomes less resonant.

EXAMINING THE RENAL SYSTEM
Palpating the kidneys

Viewed from the rear the kidneys lie in the renal angle formed by the 12th rib and the lateral margin of the vertebral column. The kidneys are not usually palpable although in thin individuals a normal-sized kidney may be felt. The right kidney lies lower than the left. Deep bimanual palpation is required to explore for them. When examining the left kidney, tuck the palmar surfaces of the left hand posteriorly into the left flank and nestle the fingertips in the renal angle. Position the middle three fingers of the right hand below the left costal margin, lateral to the rectus muscle and at a point opposite the posterior hand. To examine the right kidney, tuck your left hand behind the right loin and position the fingers of your right hand below the right costal margin, lateral to rectus abdominis. Palpate for the lower pole of each kidney in turn. Trap the lower pole of the kidney between the fingers of both hands as the organ moves up and down with deep respiration (balloting the kidney).

The kidney may be tender, especially when acutely infected (pyelonephritis) or obstructed (hydronephrosis).

It is important to distinguish kidney enlargement from splenomegaly on the left and hepatomegaly on the right. The principal cause of bilateral

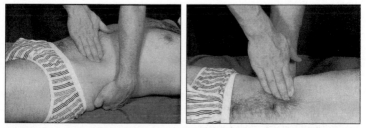

Positioning the hands when palpating (left) the left and (right) the right kidney.

Disorders
Causes of acute renal failure

- Shock (hypovolaemic, septic or cardiogenic)
- Acute glomerulonephritis
- Toxins or drugs (ethylene glycol, carbon tetrachloride)
- Acute haemoglobinuria or myoglobinuria
- Acute renal vein thrombosis

Disorders
Differentiation between splenomegaly and palpation of the left kidney

Kidney	**Enlarged spleen**
Moves late in inspiration	Moves early in inspiration
Possible to get above upper pole	Impossible to get above a spleen
Smooth shape	Notched leading edge
Resonant to percussion	Dull to percussion in Traub's space
	Enlarges towards umbilicus

Disorders
Causes of chronic renal failure

- Chronic glomerulonephritis
- Diabetes mellitus with nephropathy
- Chronic obstructive uropathy
- Polycystic disease of the kidneys
- Systemic hypertension
- Analgesic nephropathy

enlargement is polycystic disease of the kidney, whereas unilateral enlargement suggests a malignant tumour (e.g. hypernephroma).

Palpating the aorta

The aorta can be palpated between the thumb and finger of one hand or by positioning the fingers of both hands on either side of the midline at a point midway between the xiphisternum and the umbilicus.

An abdominal aortic aneurysm may be felt as a large pulsatile mass above the level of the umbilicus.

Summary
Signs of chronic renal failure

- Sallow complexion
- Anaemia (normocytic, normochromic)
- Uraemic fetor
- Deep acidotic breathing (Kussmaul respiration)
- Hypertension
- Mental clouding
- Uraemic encephalopathy (flapping tremor)

- Pleural and pericardial effusion
- Pericardial rub (pericarditis)
- Evidence of fluid overload or depletion
- Renal masses (polycystic kidneys)
- Large bladder (chronic bladder outlet obstruction)

PERCUSSION OF THE ABDOMEN
Percussion to detect ascites
In the supine position, the gas-filled normal bowel tends to float above ascites, so the gas–fluid interface characteristic of ascites is detected by a change in the percussion note from the resonance overlying bowel to the dullness of fluid. This level changes with position.

Percussion to detect a distended bladder
The suprapubic area is usually tympanic and a dull sound on percussion here is a useful clinical sign of bladder distension.

AUSCULTATION OF THE ABDOMEN
Listening for bowel sounds
Place the diaphragm of the stethoscope on the midabdomen and listen for gurgling sounds (borborygma). These peristaltic sounds occur at 5–10 second intervals, although longer silent periods may occur. Keep listening for approximately 30 seconds before concluding that bowel sounds are reduced or absent.

The absence of any bowel sounds indicate intestinal paralysis (paralytic ileus); rapidly repetitive bowel sounds (often termed 'active' bowel sounds) may be normal but they may also be an early sign of mechanical obstruction if they are associated with a colicky abdominal pain. In progressive bowel obstruction, large amounts of gas and fluid accumulate and the bowel sounds change in quality to a higher pitched 'tinkling'.

In pyloric obstruction, the stomach distends with gas and fluid; this can be detected by listening for a 'succussion splash'. Steady the diaphragm of the stethoscope on the epigastrium and shake the upper abdomen for the splashing sound characteristic of gastric outflow obstruction.

Listening for arterial bruits
Listen for renal arterial bruits at a point 2.5 cm above and lateral to the

umbilicus. The presence of a renal bruit suggests congenital or arteriosclerotic renal artery stenosis or narrowing caused by fibromuscular hyperplasia.

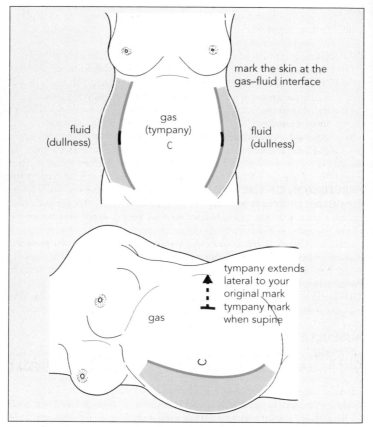

To confirm the presence of ascites, roll the patient into the right lateral position because this causes fluid to settle in the dependent right flank, whereas gas-filled bowel floats above to fill the left flank. A shift in the positions of dullness and tympany indicates free fluid.

AUSCULTATION OVER THE LIVER AND SPLEEN

Conclude the auscultation by listening over the liver and spleen. A soft and distant bruit heard over an enlarged liver is always abnormal, suggesting either primary liver cell carcinoma or acute alcoholic hepatitis. Occasionally, a creaking 'rub' may be heard over the liver or spleen. This indicates inflammation of the outer capsule of the organ.

EXAMINATION OF THE GROINS

A swelling in the groin is usually the result of either an inguinal or femoral hernia or to enlarged lymph nodes.

EXAMINING HERNIAE

An indirect inguinal hernia forms when bowel or omentum protrudes through a lax internal ring and finds its way into the inguinal canal. Bowel may force its way through the external slip into the scrotum.

An inguinal hernia usually presents as a lump in the groin or the scrotum that is most prominent when the intra-abdominal pressure is raised (e.g. when standing or coughing). It is best to examine the hernia with the patient standing. Place two fingers on the mass and ascertain whether or not an impulse is transmitted to your finger tips when the patient coughs. Most herniae can be reduced manually, so attempt this by gently massaging the mass towards the internal ring. Once the hernia is fully reduced occlude the internal ring with a finger pressing over the femoral point. Ask the patient to cough. An indirect inguinal hernia should not reappear until you release the occlusion of the internal ring.

A direct inguinal hernia develops through a weakness in the posterior wall of the inguinal canal. These herniae seldom force their way into the scrotum and, once reduced, their reappearance is not controlled by pressure over the internal ring.

When an inguinal hernia extends as far as the external ring it may be confused with a femoral hernia: an inguinal hernia lies above and medial to the tubercle, whereas a femoral hernia lies below and lateral.

EXAMINATION OF THE ANUS, RECTUM AND PROSTATE

RECTUM AND ANUS

Position the patient in the left lateral position with the hips and knees well flexed and the buttock positioned at the edge of the bed. The positions around the anal opening are described by the positions around the clock face. Gently

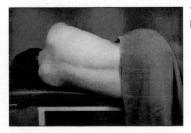

The correct position of the patient before a rectal examination.

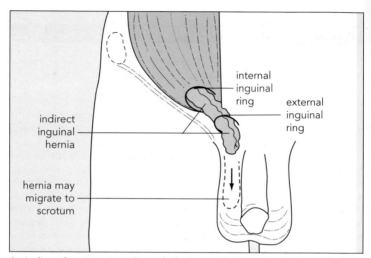

An indirect hernia enters through the internal ring and exits through the external ring.

separate the buttocks to expose the natal cleft and anal verge. Inspection may reveal skin tags, pilonidal sinuses, warts, fissures, fistulas, external haemorrhoids or prolapsed rectal mucosa. A bluish discoloration of the perineal skin disease suggests Crohn's disease.

Lubricate your index finger with a clear, water-soluble gel and press the finger tip against the anal verge with the pulp facing the 6 o'clock position. Slip your finger into the anal canal and then insert it into the rectum, directing the tip posteriorly to follow the sacral curve. Once introduced, check on anal tone.

Then gently sweep the finger through 180° using the palmar surface of the finger to explore the posterior and posterolateral walls of the rectum. Rotate the finger round to the 12 o'clock position. The normal rectum feels uniformly smooth and pliable. In men, the prostate can be felt anteriorly and in women it may be possible to feel the cervix as well as a retroverted uterus.

Withdraw your finger from the rectum and anus and check the glove tip for stool.

PROSTATE

The gland has a rubbery, smooth consistency and a shallow longitudinal groove separates the right and left lobes.

Benign hypertrophy of the prostate is smooth and symmetrical and the gland feels rubbery. A cancerous prostate may feel asymmetric, with a stony hard consistency and discrete nodules may be palpable. Marked prostatic tenderness suggests acute prostatitis, a prostatic abscess or inflammation of the seminal vesicles.

Examination of elderly people
Abdominal examination in elderly people

On inspection there may be asymmetry of the abdomen caused by kyphoscoliosis of the spine. Descent of the lower costal margin occurs with spinal osteoporosis making the abdominal examination difficult. Difficulty with hearing, comprehension or coordination may impair examination of the liver and spleen. When palpating the abdomen, the descending and sigmoid colon may be loaded with firm stool giving the impression of a left lower quadrant mass. This should be reassessed after administering an enema. An ectatic aorta may be easily palpable and spine curvature may displace the vessel to the left of the midline giving the impression of an aneurysm. Consider an aneurysm if, on palpation, you assess the aorta is greater than 5 cm in diameter at its widest. Aneurysms can be readily confirmed on abdominal ultrasound and CT scanning. Audible aortic bruits are more common in elderly people and may reflect atherosclerosis or aneurysm formation. Leakage from an aortic aneurysm may present with severe back pain and rupture presents as an acute abdominal emergency with shock, abdominal distension and poor distal perfusion with asymmetrical or absent distal pulses.

Benign and malignant prostatic hypertrophy commonly occurs in elderly men and this predisposes to bladder outlet obstruction with progressive bladder distension, urinary infection and detrusor failure. Urinary retention is a common cause of acute 'unexplained' confusion in elderly people and examination for an enlarged bladder is mandatory in all elderly patients presenting with delirium, incontinence or fever.

Faecal incontinence and constipation in elderly people
Faecal incontinence may present with or without associated urinary incontinence. Enquire about a history of constipation, diarrhoea, laxative use and bowel disease. A full neurological examination should help define central or peripheral nervous diseases and a rectal examination should help assess rectal squeeze and faecal impaction. A plain abdominal radiograph helps determine abnormal colonic loading.

Constipation (reduced stool frequency and straining at stool) is common in elderly people. The causes are similar in all age groups but in elderly patients, the disorder is most often either functional or associated with drug treatment. Enquire about previous bowel habit, duration of the disorder and, in particular, ensure you have an accurate and detailed drug history (including proprietary products such as analgesics and cough mixtures which may contain codeine). Recent onset of constipation and rectal bleeding should alert to the possibility of an organic underlying cause.

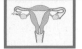

8. Female Breasts and Genitalia

SYMPTOMS OF BREAST DISEASE

PAIN
Throughout the menstrual cycle there are cyclical, trophic and involutional changes in the glandular tissue. A painful breast in the first few months of lactation is almost always due to a bacterial infection of the gland and is characterised by fever as well as redness and tenderness over the infected segment.

DISCHARGE
Determine whether the fluid is clear, opalescent or bloodstained. In men, and women who have never conceived, a discharge is always abnormal. A blood discharge should always alert you to the likelihood of an underlying breast cancer.

BREAST LUMPS
A patient may present after discovering a breast lump by self-examination.

> **⊗ Disorders**
> **Breast lumps**
>
> **Benign**
> - Fibroadenoma (mobile)
> - Simple cyst
> - Fat necrosis
> - Fibroadenosis (tender 'lumpy' breasts)
>
> - Abscess (painful and tender)
>
> **Malignant**
> - Glandular
> - Areolar

EXAMINATION OF THE BREAST

The aim of examination is to check for breast lumps and it is reasonable to recommend a formal breast examination in asymptomatic women over the age of 40 years.

INSPECTION
Position yourself in front of the patient, who should be sitting comfortably with her arms at her side. Note the size, symmetry and contour of the breasts, the colour and venous pattern of the skin. Observe the nipples and note whether they are symmetrically everted, flat or inverted. If there is unilateral flattening or nipple inversion, ask whether this is a recent or long-standing appearance. In fair-skinned women, the areola has a pink colour but darkens

and becomes permanently pigmented during the first pregnancy. Ask the patient to raise her arms above her head and then press her hands against her hips. These movements tighten the suspensory ligaments exaggerating the contours and highlighting any abnormality. In men, the nipple should lie flat on the pectoralis muscle.

ABNORMALITIES ON INSPECTION

You may be struck by an obvious lump, retraction or gross deviation of a nipple, prominent veins or oedema of the skin with dimpling like an orange skin (peau d'orange). Abnormal reddening, thickening or ulceration of the areola should alert you to the possibility of Paget's disease of the nipple.

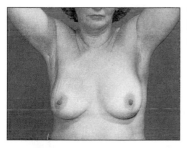

To accentuate any asymmetry of the breast ask the patient to raise her arms above her head.

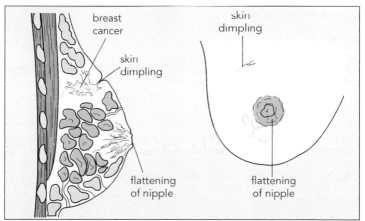

breast cancer

skin dimpling

skin dimpling

flattening of nipple

skin dimpling

flattening of nipple

Nipples may be everted, flat or retracted.

BREAST PALPATION

Palpate the breast tissue with the palmar surface of the middle three fingers, using an even rotary movement to compress the breast tissue gently towards the chest wall. Examine each breast by following a concentric or parallel trail that creates a systematic path that always begins and ends at a constant spot.

The texture of normal breast tissue varies from smooth to granular, even knotty; only experience will teach you the spectrum of normality. Remember that breast texture is normally symmetrical and a comparison of the two breasts may help you to judge whether an area is abnormal or not.

To examine the axillary tail of Spence, ask the patient to rest her arms above her head. Feel the tail between your thumb and fingers as it extends from the upper outer quadrant towards the axilla. If you feel a breast lump, examine the mass between your fingers and assess its size, consistency, mobility and whether or not there is any tenderness.

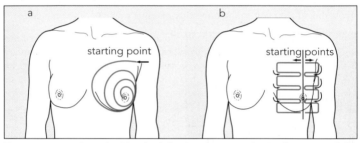

Trace a systematic path either by following a concentric circular pattern (left) or examining each half of the breast sequentially from above down (right).

NIPPLE PALPATION

Hold the nipple between thumb and fingers and gently compress and attempt to express any discharge. If fluid appears, note its colour, prepare a smear for cytology and send a swab for microbiology.

LYMPH NODE PALPATION

The axillae can be palpated with the patient lying or sitting. When examining the left axilla in the sitting position, the patient may rest her (or his) left hand on your right shoulder while you explore the axilla with your right hand. Feel for the anterior group of nodes along the posterior border of the anterior axillary fold, the central group against the lateral chest wall and the posterior group along the posterior axillary fold. Finally, palpate along the medial border of the humerus to check for the lateral group of nodes and inspect the infraclavicular and supraclavicular spaces for lymphadenopathy. If you feel nodes, assess the size, shape, consistency, mobility and tenderness.

ABNORMAL PALPATION
Breast lumps

Common benign lumps include fibroadenomas, fibroadenosis, benign breast cysts and fat necrosis. Cancerous lesions usually feel hard and irregular and, unlike benign lesions, may be fixed to the skin or the underlying chest wall muscle.

Breast abscess (mastitis)

This usually occurs during lactation and is generally caused by blockage of a duct. The temperature is raised and the skin of the infected breasts inflamed. Palpation may reveal an area of tenderness and induration. If an abscess forms, you usually feel an extremely tender fluctuant mass.

Abnormal nipple and areola

A bloodstained nipple discharge suggests an intraductal carcinoma or benign papilloma. Unilateral retraction or distortion of a nipple should also alert you to the possibility of malignancy. Blockage of the sebaceous glands of Montgomery may cause retention cysts.

Palpable lymph nodes

If you detect axillary lymphadenopathy, suspect malignancy if the nodes are hard, nontender or fixed. Infection of axillary hair follicles or breast tissue may cause tender lymphadenitis.

Summary
Breast examination

Inspection
- Symmetry and contour
- Venous pattern of skin
- Nipples (asymmetry, inversion)
- Areola (chloasma, skin ulceration, thickening)

Breast palpation
- Texture
- Symmetry

- Tenderness
- Masses (mobility, size)
- Tail of Spence

Lymph node palpation
- Axillary nodes (five groups)
- Contralateral axillary nodes
- Infraclavicular and supraclavicular nodes

SYMPTOMS OF GENITAL TRACT DISEASE

MENSTRUAL HISTORY
Establish the age of the menarche

By the age of 14 years, secondary sexual characteristics should have appeared. If the menarche has not occurred and there are no other signs of sexual development, it is reasonable to consider organic causes of primary amenorrhoea, such as gonadal dysgenesis (Turner's syndrome), congenital anatomical abnormalities of the genital tract, polycystic ovaries or pituitary or hypothalamic tumours in childhood. If secondary sexual characteristics have appeared, investigation is usually only necessary if the menarche has not occurred by the age of 16 years.

Determine the pattern of the menstrual cycle

Attempt to classify any change or abnormality in the menstrual cycle. The most common irregularities include failure to menstruate at the expected time (secondary amenorrhoea). Cycles may be infrequent and scanty (oligomenorrhoea), unusually frequent (polymenorrhoea), excessively heavy (menorrhagia) or frequent and heavy (polymenorrhagia). Bleeding after intercourse is termed postcoital bleeding.

Questions to ask
The menstrual cycle

- Age of menarche?
- Age of telarche?
- Do you use the contraceptive pill or hormone replacement therapy?
- Length of cycle?
- Days of blood loss?
- Number of tampons or pads used per day?
- Are there clots?
- Has there been a change in the periodicity of the cycle?

Secondary amenorrhoea

Pregnancy and lactation are the most common causes.

Disorders
Causes of secondary amenorrhoea

Physiological
- Pregnancy
- Lactation

Psychological
- Anorexia nervosa
- Depression
- Fear of pregnancy

Hormonal
- Postcontraceptive pill
- Pituitary tumours

- Hyperthyroidism
- Adrenal tumours

Ovarian
- Polycystic ovaries
- Ovarian tumour
- Ovarian tuberculosis
- Constitutional disease
- Severe acute illness
- Chronic infections or illnesses
- Autoimmune diseases

Abnormal patterns of uterine bleeding
Oligomenorrhoea
Infrequent or scanty menstrual periods. If oligomenorrhoea presents as a distinct change in the menstrual pattern, consider the same factors implicated in the differential diagnosis of secondary amenorrhoea.

Dysfunctional uterine bleeding
Frequent bleeding or excessive menstrual loss that cannot be ascribed to local pelvic pathology (e.g. fibroids, pelvic inflammatory disease, carcinoma, polyps). Regular dysfunctional bleeding implies that ovulation is occurring. Irregular dysfunctional bleeding usually implies that ovulation has ceased; the menstrual rhythm is lost and the cyclical pattern is replaced by unpredictable bleeding of varying severity.

Intermenstrual and postmenopausal bleeding
Diseases of the uterus and cervix may present with abnormal bleeding, so consider disorders of the mucosa or submucosa. Postcoital bleeding usually indicates local cervical or uterine disease (carcinoma or a cervical polyp).

Vaginal discharge
A physiological discharge is scanty, mucoid and odourless. Pathological discharge is usually trichomonal or candidal vaginitis. The discharge may irritate the vulval skin causing itching (pruritus vulvae) or burning.

Questions to ask
Vaginal discharge

- How long has the discharge been present?
- Is the discharge scanty or profuse?
- Is extra protection necessary or does the discharge simply spot or stain?
- What is the colour and consistency?
- Is there an odour?
- Is the discharge bloodstained?
- Is there associated lower abdominal pain and fever?
- Is there itching or burning of the vulval area?

Pain
If the pain predictably occurs immediately before and during a period, the likely cause is dysmenorrhoea. Severe dysmenorrhoea should alert you to the possibility of endometriosis.

Ovulation may cause a unilateral iliac fossa or suprapubic pain in midcycle which lasts a few hours (mittleschmertz). Severe iliac fossa pain should warn

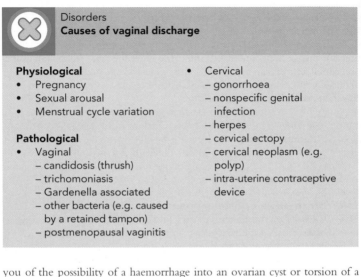

Disorders
Causes of vaginal discharge

Physiological
- Pregnancy
- Sexual arousal
- Menstrual cycle variation

Pathological
- Vaginal
  - candidosis (thrush)
  - trichomoniasis
  - Gardenella associated
  - other bacteria (e.g. caused by a retained tampon)
  - postmenopausal vaginitis

- Cervical
  - gonorrhoea
  - nonspecific genital infection
  - herpes
  - cervical ectopy
  - cervical neoplasm (e.g. polyp)
  - intra-uterine contraceptive device

you of the possibility of a haemorrhage into an ovarian cyst or torsion of a cyst. If the pain is preceded by a missed period and especially if there is shock, you should also consider the possibility of a ruptured ectopic pregnancy. If the lower abdominal pain is accompanied by a vaginal discharge, fever, anorexia and nausea, consider acute infection of the fallopian tubes (acute salpingitis).

Dyspareunia

Pain on intercourse (dyspareunia) may be caused by either psychological or organic disorders. Assess whether the pain is superficial (suggesting a local vulval cause or a psychological spasm) or deep (suggesting inflammatory or malignant disease of the cervix, uterus or adnexae).

Psychosexual history

Questions to ask
Psychosexual history

- Are you able to develop satisfying emotional relationships?
- Do you have satisfying physical relationships?
- Are you heterosexual, homosexual or ambivalent?
- Do you use contraception and, if so, what form?
- Do you have problems achieving arousal?
- Do you experience orgasm?

OBSTETRIC HISTORY

Enquire whether the patient has ever been pregnant and whether there were fertility problems. Record the number of completed and unsuccessful pregnancies. If the patient has miscarried, record the maturity of the pregnancy at the time of miscarriage. Ask about complications during pregnancy (e.g. hypertension, diabetes) and problems associated with labour and the period after delivery (the puerperium).

Questions to ask
Obstetric history

- Have you ever been pregnant and, if so, how often?
- Did you have any problems falling pregnant?
- How many children do you have?
- Have you miscarried and, if so, at what stage of pregnancy?
- Were there any complications in pregnancy (e.g. high blood pressure or diabetes)?
- Was the labour normal or did you require forceps assistance or a caesarean section?

EXAMINATION OF THE FEMALE GENITAL TRACT

GENERAL EXAMINATION

Before examining the genital tract you should perform a general examination.

EXAMINATION OF THE ABDOMEN

A full abdominal examination precedes the vulval and vaginal examination. Although the uterus and adnexae lie deep within the protective confines of the pelvis, abnormalities may be apparent above the pubis. Lower abdominal tenderness occurs in pelvic inflammatory disease and enlargement of the uterus or ovaries may present with a palpable lower abdominal mass. Large ovarian cysts may fill the abdomen; this presentation is readily mistaken for ascites. Careful abdominal percussion helps distinguish ascites from a cystic ovarian tumour. A large ovarian cyst displaces the bowel laterally and on percussion there is central dullness with resonance in the flanks. This contrasts with ascites which is characterised by central resonance and dullness in the flanks.

Abdomen in pregnancy

After the 12th week of the pregnancy, the uterus becomes palpable above the symphysis pubis, making it possible to assess the maturity of the foetus from the height of the fundus.

EXAMINATION OF THE EXTERNAL GENITALIA

The patient lies supine with the hips and knees flexed and the heels close together. When examining the vulva and vagina, wear disposable plastic gloves on each hand.

INSPECTION AND PALPATION OF THE VULVA

The pattern of hair distribution over the mons pubis provides a useful measure of sexual development. Gently separate the labia with the fingers of your left hand and inspect the medial aspect which should be pink and slightly moist. Palpate the length of the labia majora between index finger and thumb; the tissue should feel pliant and fleshy. Next, examine the Bartholin's gland between the index finger and thumb. The right index finger palpates from the entrance of the vagina while the thumb palpates the outer surface of the labia majora posteriorly. A normal Bartholin's gland is not palpable.

To expose the vestibule, separate the labia minora. The vestibular tissue should be supple and slightly moist. Separation of the labia minora exposes the vaginal orifice and urethra.

Abnormalities of the vulva

A confluent, itchy, red rash on the inner aspects of the thighs and extending to the labia suggests candidiasis. A vaginal discharge due to candidiasis or a trichomonal infection may irritate the vulval skin causing redness and tenderness (vulvitis).

The vulva is a common site for boils (furuncles) to appear. These are tender to palpation and should be distinguished from sebaceous cysts which are firm, rounded, yellowish and nontender, with an apical punctum indicating the opening of the blocked duct.

Crops of small, painful, vulval and perianal papules and vesicles that ulcerate suggest a herpes simplex infection. Flat, round or oval papules covered by a grey exudate suggests lesions of secondary syphilis (condylomata latum).

Acute vulval ulceration occurring with mouth and tongue ulcers and inflamed red eyes suggests Behçet's syndrome. A firm painless labial ulcer suggests the chancre of primary syphilis, whereas broad, moist ulcerating papules covered by grey slough suggest secondary syphilis.

Leukoplakia is a potentially malignant, hypertrophic skin lesion affecting the labia, clitoris and perineum. The skin thickens, feels hard and indurated and is distinguished from surrounding tissue by its white colour.

Bartholin's glands are palpable if the ducts obstruct. This results in a painless cystic mass or an acute (Bartholin's) abscess: a hot, red, tender swelling in the posterolateral labia majora deep to the posterior end of the labia minora.

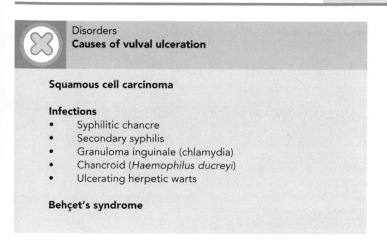

Disorders
Causes of vulval ulceration

Squamous cell carcinoma

Infections
- Syphilitic chancre
- Secondary syphilis
- Granuloma inguinale (chlamydia)
- Chancroid (*Haemophilus ducreyi*)
- Ulcerating herpetic warts

Behçet's syndrome

EXAMINATION OF THE VAGINA

A full vaginal examination includes inspection with a speculum, followed by a bimanual examination of the uterus and adnexae.

SPECULUM EXAMINATION

Warm the blades under a stream of tepid water. Use the index and middle fingers of the free hand to separate the labia and expose the introitus.

EXAMINATION OF THE CERVIX

The cervix usually points posteriorly and the uterus lies in an anterior plane (anteversion). Conversely, the cervix may point anteriorly with the uterus in a posterior retroverted position. There are also intermediate positions between these two. The shape of the external os changes after childbirth. In nulliparous women, the os is round, whereas after childbirth, the os may be slit-like or stellate.

Inspect the colour of the cervix. The surface of the cervix is pink, smooth and regular, and resembles the epithelium of the vagina. In early pregnancy the cervix has a bluish colour caused by increased vascularity (Chadwick's sign). Cervical 'erosions' are not ulcerated surfaces but a term used to describe the appearance of the cervix when the endocervical epithelium extends onto the outer surface of the cervix. The columnar epithelium appears as a strawberry-red area spreading circumferentially around the os or onto the anterior or posterior lips.

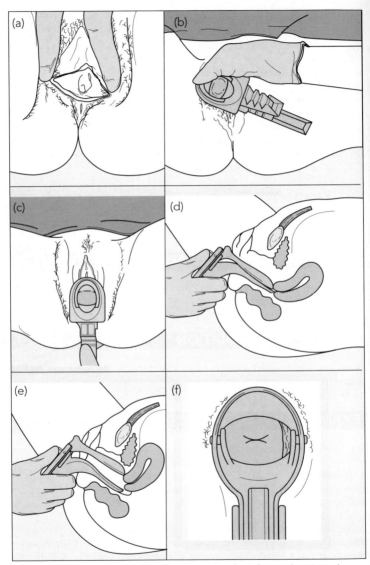

(a) Expose the vaginal opening, (b) direct the closed speculum into the vagina, (c) rotate the speculum as it penetrates the long axis. (d) Final position of the fully inserted speculum. (e) Open the blades. (f) Search for the cervix and os.

ABNORMALITIES OF THE CERVIX

Nabothian cysts may develop if there is obstruction of the endocervical glands. There may be a cervical discharge. If there is a pungent odour, suspect an infective cause. An inflamed cervix covered by a mucopurulent discharge or slough is characteristic of acute and chronic cervicitis. Cherry-red friable polyps may grow from the cervix (a source of vaginal bleeding after intercourse). Ulceration and fungating growths suggest cervical carcinoma.

Cervical smear

Cytologists can detect premalignant cells or established cervical cancer by examining a preparation of cells scraped from the surface of the cervix.

INTERNAL EXAMINATION OF THE UTERUS

The speculum examination is followed by the vaginal examination. Again, expose the introitus by separating the labia with the thumb and forefinger of the gloved left hand and gently introduce the gloved and lubricated right index and middle fingers into the vagina, remembering that the organ is directed backwards in the direction of the sacrum. Palpate the vaginal wall as you introduce your fingers. The walls are slightly rugose, supple and moist.

CERVIX

Locate the cervix with the pulps of your fingertips. The cervix should feel firm, rounded and smooth. Assess the mobility of the cervix by moving it gently and palpate the fornices.

Abnormalities of the cervix

In pregnancy, the cervix softens (Hegar's sign). If there is tenderness on movement (known as 'excitation tenderness'), suspect infection or inflammation of the uterus or adnexae; or if the patient is shocked, suspect an ectopic pregnancy. You may palpate an ulcer or tumour already noted on the speculum examination.

UTERUS

Next, palpate the uterus. A bimanual technique is used to assess the size and position of the organ.

Abnormalities of the uterus

If the uterus appears to be uniformly enlarged, consider a pregnancy, fibroid or endometrial tumour. Fibromyomas (fibroids) are common benign uterine tumours which may be single or multiple and may vary in size.

ADNEXAE

Palpate the left and right adnexae in turn. Place the fingers of your abdominal hand over the iliac fossa whilst readjusting the vaginal fingers into the lateral

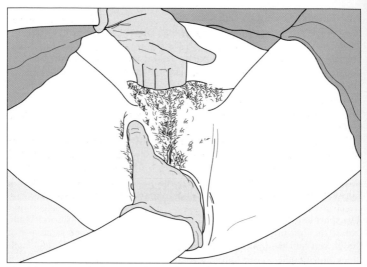

The bimanual technique used to palpate the uterus. The vaginal fingers lift the cervix, while the other hand dips downwards and inwards to meet the fundus.

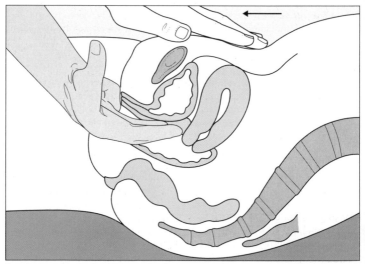

By placing the vaginal fingers in the anterior fornix it is possible to examine the anterior surface of the uterus.

fornix and positioning the finger pulps to face the abdominal fingers. Remembering the anatomy of the ovaries and fallopian tubes, gently but firmly appose the fingers of either hand by pressing the abdominal hand inward and downward, and the vaginal fingers upwards and laterally. Feel for the adnexal structures as the interposed tissues slip between your fingers.

Abnormalities of the adnexal structures

The most common causes of enlarged ovaries include benign cysts (e.g. follicular or corpus luteal cysts) and malignant ovarian tumours.

In acute infections of the fallopian tubes (salpingitis), there is lower abdominal tenderness and guarding, and on vaginal examination, marked tenderness of the lateral fornices and cervix. In chronic salpingitis, the lower abdomen and lateral fornices are tender, yet the uterus and adnexae may be amenable to examination. If the tubes are blocked, there may be cystic swelling of the tubes (hydrosalpinx) or they may become infected and purulent (pyosalpinx).

Examination of elderly people
Breasts and genital tract

The menopause is associated with a rapid fall in sex hormone synthesis and this results in rapid and significant alterations in the breasts and genitalia. The postmenopausal period is characterised by progressive involution of breast tissue and the breasts often become pendulous as acinar tissue atrophies. The breast remains susceptible to cancer at all ages including the very aged. After the menopause, there is loss of vulval adipose tissue, vaginal secretion is markedly reduced and there is general atrophy of the tissue of the introitus with narrowing of the vestibule and an increased susceptibility to ascending urinary tract infection. The loss of female sex hormones also results in altered hair distribution and in elderly women an androgenic dominance may be apparent with male-pattern facial hair growth, mild to moderate male-pattern hair loss and loss of labial hair.

Despite the involutional changes, many women maintain their libido and remain sexually active well into the later years of life and an active sexual interest by elderly people is normal behaviour. Atrophy of the introitus and vagina can be prevented by hormone replacement therapy and topical oestrogen treatment and lubrication of the vagina can be enhanced by using lubricant jelly.

9. The Male Genitalia

SYMPTOMS OF GENITAL TRACT DISEASE

URETHRAL DISCHARGE

Questions to ask
Urethral discharge

- Is there a possibility of recent exposure to a sexually transmitted disease?
- How long ago might you have had such a contact (incubation period)?
- Does your partner complain of a vaginal discharge?
- Have you experienced joint pains or gritty, red eyes?
- Have you recently suffered from gastroenteritis?

Disorders
Causes of urethral discharge

Physiological
- Sexual arousal

Pathological
- Gonococcal urethritis (incubation period 2–6 days)
- Nongonococcal urethritis
- Idiopathic nonspecific urethritis
- *Chlamydia trachomatis*
- *Trichomonas vaginalis*
- *Candida albicans*
- Posturinary catheter
- Reiter's syndrome (may follow gastroenteritis) includes arthritis and conjunctivitis

GENITAL ULCERS

The appearance of an ulcer or 'sore' always raises the spectre of venereal disease. Herpetic ulcers tend to recur and may be preceded by a prodrome of a prickly sensation or pain in the loins.

TESTICULAR PAIN

Inflammation or trauma to the testes causes an intense visceral pain that may radiate towards the groin and abdomen.

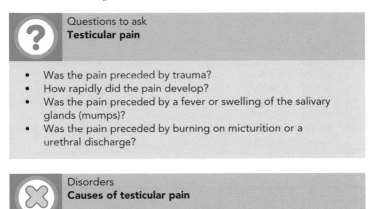

Questions to ask
Testicular pain

- Was the pain preceded by trauma?
- How rapidly did the pain develop?
- Was the pain preceded by a fever or swelling of the salivary glands (mumps)?
- Was the pain preceded by burning on micturition or a urethral discharge?

Disorders
Causes of testicular pain

- Trauma
- Infection (mumps orchitis)
- Epididymitis
- Testicular torsion
- Torsion of epididymal cyst

IMPOTENCE

Impotence is often a manifestation of emotional disturbance, therefore, you should try to assess whether the patient is depressed, anxious about sexual encounters or troubled by emotional aspects of the relationship. An obvious association with organic disease may be apparent in patients presenting with concomitant cardiovascular, respiratory or neurological symptoms.

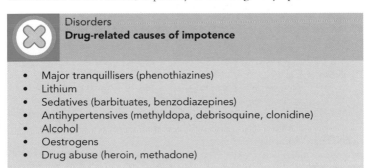

Disorders
Drug-related causes of impotence

- Major tranquillisers (phenothiazines)
- Lithium
- Sedatives (barbituates, benzodiazepines)
- Antihypertensives (methyldopa, debrisoquine, clonidine)
- Alcohol
- Oestrogens
- Drug abuse (heroin, methadone)

INFERTILITY

Questions to ask
Infertility

- Have you or your partner ever conceived?
- Do you have difficulty obtaining or maintaining an erection?
- Do you ejaculate?
- Do you understand the timing of ovulation in your partner?
- Are you on any medication that may cause impotence or sperm malfunction (e.g. salazopyrine)?
- Have you noticed any change in facial hair growth?
- Have you ever had cancer treatment?

GENERAL EXAMINATION OF THE MALE GENITALIA

You will already have performed a general examination and noted the distribution of facial, axillary and abdominal hair. In testicular malfunction (hypogonadism), there may be loss of axillary hair, the pubic hair distribution may start to resemble the distinctive female pattern and there is a typical facial appearance with wrinkling around the mouth. You will have also checked the breast and noted whether or not gynaecomastia is evident.

Disorders
Causes of male gynaecomastia

Physiological
- Puberty
- Old age

Pathological
- Hypogonadism
- Liver cirrhosis
- Drugs (spironolactone, digoxin, oestrogens)
- Tumours (bronchogenic carcinoma, adrenal carcinoma, testicular tumours)
- Thyrotoxicosis

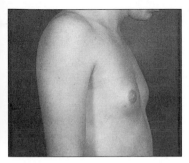

Typical appearance of male gynaecomastia.

NORMAL PENIS

The length and thickness of the flaccid penis vary widely and bear no relationship either to potency or to fertility. The dorsal vein of the penis is usually prominent along the dorsal midline. Gently retract the foreskin (prepuce) to expose the glans penis. The foreskin should be supple, allowing smooth and painless retraction. There is often a trace of odourless, curd-like smegma underlying the foreskin. Examine the external urethral meatus which is a slit-like orifice extending from the ventral pole of the tip of the glans. Use your index finger and thumb to squeeze the meatus gently open. This should expose healthy, glistening pink mucosa.

Abnormalities of the penis
Prepuce
The prepuce may be too tight to retract over the glans (phimosis). If the prepuce is tight but retracts and catches behind the glans, oedema and swelling may occur, preventing the return of the foreskin (paraphimosis)

Glans
Hypospadias is a developmental abnormality causing the urethral meatus to appear on the inferior (ventral) surface of the glans.

Urethral discharge
This is one of the most common genital disorders in men and is caused by urethral inflammation (urethritis).

Penile ulcers
The most common cause is herpetic ulceration.

Priapism
A painful and prolonged erection is termed priapism. Most often there is no obvious cause but predisposing factors such as leukaemia, haemo-globinopathies (e.g. sickle cell anaemia) and drugs (aphrodisiacs) should be considered.

Disorders
Causes of genital ulcers

Infections
- Genital herpes
- Syphilis (chancre, mucous patches, gumma)
- Tropical ulcers

Balanitis
- Severe candida
- Circinate balanitis (Reiter's syndrome)

Drug eruption
- Localised fixed drug eruption
- Generalised (Stevens–Johnson syndrome)

Carcinoma
- Behçet's syndrome

EXAMINATION OF THE SCROTUM

The left testis lies lower than the right. Ensure that your hands are warm before palpating the testis. Use gentle pressure, sufficient to explore the bulk of the tissue without causing pain. Compare the left and right testes because many testicular disorders are unilateral. Feel the testicle between your thumb and first two fingers. Note the size and consistency of the testis. Next, palpate the epididymis which is felt as an elongated structure along the posterolateral surface of the testicle. Finally, roll with the finger and thumb the vas deferens which passes from the tail of the epididymis to the inguinal canal through the external inguinal canal.

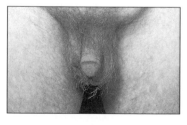

The left testis lies lower than the right.

Abnormalities of the scrotum
Scrotum

If one-half of the scrotum appears smooth and poorly developed, consider an undescended testis (cryptorchidism).

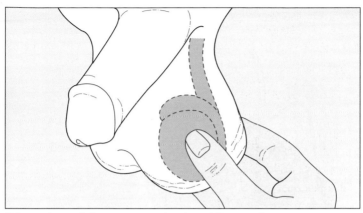

Palpate the testis between your thumb and first two fingers.

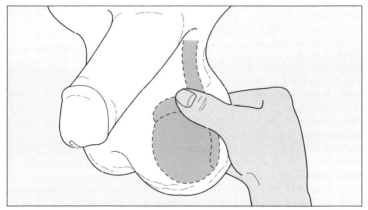

The epididymis is felt along the posterior pole of the testis.

Swellings in the scrotum
Decide whether the swelling arises from an indirect inguinal hernia or from the scrotal contents. It is possible to 'get above' a testicular swelling but not a scrotal hernia.

Cystic swelling
Cystic accumulations are caused by entrapment of fluid in the tunica vaginalis (a hydrocoele) or accumulation of fluid in an epididymal cyst, and are typically fluctuant. Cystic lesions usually transilluminate. An epididymal cyst is felt as a distinct swelling behind the adjoining testis. In contrast, a hydro-coele surrounds and envelops the testis which becomes impalpable as a discreet organ.

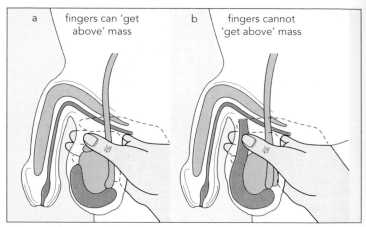

It is possible to 'get above' a true scrotal swelling (a), whereas this is not possible if the swelling is caused by an inguinal hernia that has descended into the scrotum (b).

Varicocoele

A varicocoele results from a varicosity of the veins of the pampiniform plexus, a leash of vessels surrounding the spermatic cord, and is caused by abnormality of the valve mechanism of the left testicular vein which drains into the left renal vein. Examine the patient in the standing position; the varicocoele feels like a 'bag of worms'. A characteristic feature is transmission of the raised intra-abdominal pressure to the varicocoele which is felt as a discreet cough impulse. A varicocoele usually empties when the patient lies supine.

Solid swellings

Diffuse, acutely painful swelling usually occurs in acute inflammatory condition such as orchitis or torsion of the testis. Solid masses may be smooth or craggy, tender or painless but, whatever the character, carcinoma must be the first differential diagnosis. Other solid masses include tuberculomas and syphilitic gummas. Solid tumours of the epididymis are due to chronic inflammation (usually tuberculous epididymitis).

Torsion of the testis

This usually occurs in young boys and presents with severe scrotal pain. The affected testis lies higher than the unaffected testis. The testis may be very tender and the spermatic cord may feel thickened and sensitive to palpation.

Scrotal oedema

Scrotal oedema usually occurs when there is diffuse oedema (anasarca) caused by severe congestive heart failure or nephrotic syndrome.

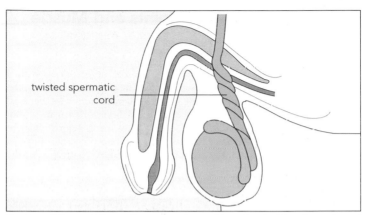

twisted spermatic cord

Torsion of the testicle on the spermatic cord impairs the blood supply. The affected testis is swollen and tender and lies higher than expected. The overlying scrotal skin is often reddened and oedematous.

EXAMINATION OF THE LYMPHATICS
The skin lymphatics of the penis and scrotum drain towards the inguinal nodes; you should complete your genital examination by feeling for nodes in the groin which are felt deep to the inguinal crease. The testicular lymphatics drain to intra-abdominal nodes.

Enlarged inguinal nodes
Enlarged nodes occur in infective and malignant disorders affecting the skin of the penis and scrotum. The primary chancre of syphilis is usually associated with lymphadenopathy. The nodes are typically mobile, rubbery and not tender.

Examination of elderly people
Genitalia of elderly people

Men may remain sexually active throughout life, although impotence and loss of libido are common in elderly men, especially when illness or infirmity supervenes. There is no male equivalent of the female menopause and whereas most women have lost ovarian function by 50 years of age, most men continue to produce sperm into the eighth and even ninth decades. Benign prostatic hypertrophy causes prostatism in most elderly men and, although this does not affect genital function, prostatectomy often results in retrograde ejaculation. Hydrocoele and varicocoele are common causes of testicular swelling in elderly men but cancer of the testis usually occurs in young men.

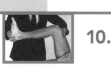

10. Bone, Joints and Muscle

The skeleton provides protection for the internal organs along with a strengthening and support system for the limbs. The presence of joints in the limbs and spine permits movement of what would otherwise be rigid structures. The cartilage interposed between the bone surfaces of a joint cushions the forces that are generated during movement. Joint strength is enhanced by ligaments that are either incorporated into the joint capsule or independent of it. Movement at the joint is achieved by contraction of the muscles passing across it.

SYMPTOMS OF BONE. JOINT AND MUSCLE DISORDERS

BONE
Pain
Bone pain has a deep, boring quality. The pain is focal in the presence of a bone tumour or infection but diffuse in generalised disorders (e.g. osteoporosis). The pain of a fracture is sharp and piercing and exacerbated by movement but relieved by rest.

Disorders
Causes of bone pain

Focal pain	**Diffuse pain**
• Fracture or trauma	• Malignancy
• Infection	• Paget's disease
• Malignancy	• Osteomalacia
• Paget's disease	• Osteoporosis
• Osteoid osteoma	• Metabolic bone disease

JOINTS
Joint symptoms include pain, swelling, crepitus and locking.

Pain
In an arthritic disorder, pain is usually the most prominent complaint. Important aspects to determine are the site and severity of the pain, whether it is acute or chronic, how it is influenced by rest and activity and whether it appears during a particular range of movement.

The segments to which the pain is referred (the sclerotomes) differ somewhat from dermatomal distributions. Consequently, deep pain can be felt at a point some distance from the affected structure, that is, referred pain. Where joint disease exists, misinterpretation of the site of the disease process can follow. Osteoarthritis and rheumatoid arthritis typically result in chronic pain with periodic exacerbation; septic arthritis or gout produce an acute, very painful joint.

Inflammatory joint disease tends to cause pain on waking, improving with activity but returning at rest. Mechanical joint disease (e.g. caused by osteoarthritis) leads to pain that worsens during the course of the day, particularly with activity.

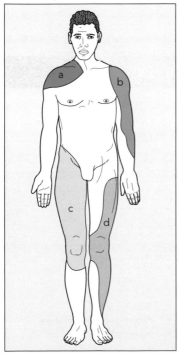

Distribution of pain arising from (a) the acromioclavicular or sternoclavicular joints, (b) the scapulohumeral joint, (c) the hip joint and (d) the knee joint.

Questions to ask
Joint pain

- Where is the maximal site of pain?
- Does the pain change during the course of the day?
- Has the pain been there for a short or long time?
- Does the pain get better or worse as you move about?

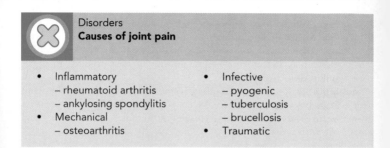

Disorders
Causes of joint pain

- Inflammatory
  - rheumatoid arthritis
  - ankylosing spondylitis
- Mechanical
  - osteoarthritis
- Infective
  - pyogenic
  - tuberculosis
  - brucellosis
- Traumatic

Swelling and crepitus
If the patient has noticed joint swelling, elicit for how long it has been present, whether there is associated pain and whether the swelling fluctuates. A noisy joint is not necessarily pathological. Crepitus is a grating noise or sensation; it can have both auditory and palpable qualities.

Locking
A joint locks if ectopic material becomes interposed between the articular surfaces. It is particularly associated with damage to the knee cartilages.

MUSCLE
Muscle symptoms include pain and stiffness, weakness, wasting, abnormal spontaneous movements and cramps.

Pain and stiffness
Muscle pain tends to be deep, constant and poorly localised.

Disorders
Causes of muscle pain

- Inflammatory
  - polymyositis
  - dermatomyositis
- Infective
  - pyogenic
  - cysticercosis
- Traumatic
- Polymyalgia rheumatica
- Neuropathic
  - e.g. Guillain–Barré
    syndrome

Weakness
Important questions to ask include the distribution of the weakness, whether it appears related to any pain in the limb, whether it fluctuates and whether it is static or progressive.

Questions to ask
Muscle weakness

- Is the weakness global or focal?
- Is the weakness secondary to a painful limb?
- Does the weakness fluctuate?
- Is the weakness increasing in severity?

Wasting and fasciculation

If the patient describes muscle twitching, ascertain whether the movement has occurred in several different muscles or whether it has been confined to one area, most likely the calf.

Cramps

Cramps are seldom of pathological significance. They are usually confined to the calves and can be triggered by forced contraction of the muscle.

GENERAL PRINCIPLES OF EXAMINATION

INSPECTION

Things you are looking for include swelling, joint deformity, overlying skin changes and the appearance of the surrounding structures.

Swelling

Causes of joint swelling include effusions and thickening of the synovial tissues and bony margins of the joint.

Deformity

Deformity results either from misalignment of the bones forming the joint or from alteration of the relationship between the articular surfaces. If misalignment exists, a deviation of the part distal to the joint away from the midline is called a valgus deformity and a deviation towards the midline a varus deformity. Partial loss of contact of the articulating surfaces is called subluxation and complete loss, dislocation. Swan neck, Boutonnière and mallet are descriptive terms used for deformities of the metacarpophalangeal and interphalangeal joints of the hand.

Skin changes

Redness of the skin over a joint implies an underlying acute inflammatory reaction (e.g. gout).

Changes of adjacent structures

The most striking change adjacent to a diseased joint is wasting of muscle.

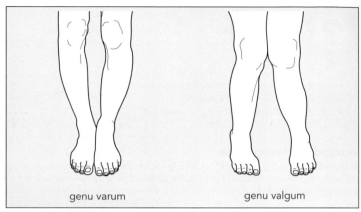

Genu varum (left) and genu valgum (right).

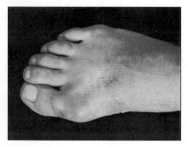

Acute gout of the first metatarsophalangeal joint

PALPATION

During palpation of a joint, assess the nature of any swelling, whether there is tenderness and whether the joint is hot.

Swelling

Your first step is to determine the consistency of any swelling. Is the swelling hard, suggesting bone deformities secondary to osteoarthritis? A slightly spongy or boggy swelling suggests synovial thickening and is particularly associated with rheumatoid arthritis. An effusion is fluctuant, that is, the fluid can be displaced from one part of the joint to another.

Tenderness

Carefully palpate the joint margin and adjacent bony surfaces together with the surrounding ligaments and tendons. In an acutely inflamed joint, the whole of its palpable contours will be tender. If there is derangement of a single knee cartilage, tenderness will be confined to the margin of that cartilage.

Temperature

For a small joint, for example, in the finger, assess temperature with the finger tips, using an unaffected joint in the same or the other hand for comparison. For a larger joint, for example, the knee, rub the back of your hand across the joint then compare with the other limb.

Movement

To define the range of joint movement, start with the joints in the neutral position, defined as the limbs extended with the feet dorsi-flexed to 90°, the upper limbs midway between pronation and supination with the arms flexed to 90° at the elbows. Movement of a joint is either active (i.e. induced by the patient) or passive (i.e. induced by the examiner).

From the neutral position, record the degrees of flexion and extension. If extension does not normally occur at a joint (e.g. the knee) but is present, describe the movement as hyperextension and give its range in degrees.

MUSCLE

Initially your assessment will include inspection, palpation, then testing of muscle power.

Inspection

Look for evidence of muscle wasting, for signs of abnormal muscle bulk and for spontaneous contractions.

Wasting

If there is no significant joint disease, wasting (other than caused by a profound loss of body weight) reflects either primary muscle disease or disease of its innervating neuron.

Increased muscle bulk

There are rare conditions that lead to muscle hypertrophy. If the enlargement is due to increase in muscle bulk, it is called true hypertrophy and is seen, for example, in congenital myotonia. If the increased bulk is due to fatty infiltration (and you will then discover the muscle is actually weak) it is called pseudohypertrophy.

Spontaneous contractions

Spontaneous contractions can occur with both upper and lower motor neuron lesions. In the former, particularly at the spinal level, you may see either flexor or extensor spasms of the legs, either at the hips or knees. Fasciculation produces episodic muscle twitching that can be subtle in small muscles. It is a feature of lower motor neuron lesions but can also be seen in normal individuals.

Palpation

Muscle palpation is of limited value.

Testing muscle power

You should follow the UK Medical Research Council classification when testing and recording muscle power. If muscle fatigue is a prominent symptom, assess it objectively. For example, for the deltoid, ask the patient to abduct the shoulder to 90° then, test power immediately after the patient has held that posture for 60 s.

REGIONAL STRUCTURE, FUNCTION AND EXAMINATION

TEMPOROMANDIBULAR JOINTS

Ask the patient to open and close the jaw. If the temporomandibular joints are lax, there may be considerable side-to-side movement. Now palpate the joint margins by placing your fingers immediately in front of and below the tragus.

EXAMINATION OF THE SPINE

Assess the posture of the whole spine before examining its component parts. An increased flexion is called kyphosis, increased extension is lordosis and a lateral curvature is scoliosis. Gibbus refers to a focal flexion deformity.

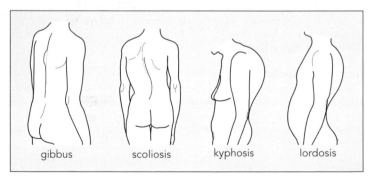

gibbus   scoliosis   kyphosis   lordosis

Spinal deformities.

CERVICAL SPINE

The examination is best achieved with the patient sitting. Note any deformity, then palpate the spinous processes.

Examine active then passive movements. Note whether any movement triggers pain either locally or in the upper limb.

THORACIC SPINE
Sit the patient with his or her arms folded across the chest, then ask the patient to twist as far as possible first to one side then to the other. The range of movement is best appreciated from above. Next measure chest expansion.

LUMBAR SPINE
Having inspected the lumbar spine and tested for tenderness, assess the range of movement.

SACRO-ILIAC JOINTS
Palpate the joints, which lie under the dimples found in the lower lumbar region. To test whether movement at the joint is painful, first press firmly down over the midline of the sacrum with the patient prone then, with the patient supine, forcibly flex one hip while maintaining the other in an extended position.

NERVE STRETCH TESTS
Nerve stretch tests are carried out to determine whether there is evidence of nerve root irritation, usually as a consequence of prolapse of a lumbar disc.

Femoral stretch test

(a) Femoral stretch. The pain may be triggered by (b) knee flexion alone or (c) in combination with hip extension.

Straight leg raising

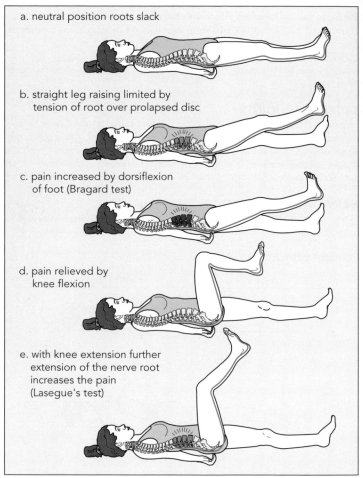

Stretch tests: (a) neutral position, (b) straight leg raising, (c) Bragard's test, (d) knee flexion) and (e) Lasegue's test.

CLINICAL APPLICATION

PROLAPSED INTERVERTEBRAL DISC

A prolapse of disc material is most likely to occur either in the cervical (principally at C5/6) or the lumbar (principally at L5/S1) region.

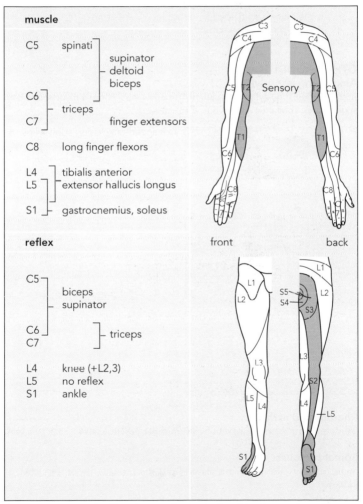

Sensory, motor and reflex changes in cervical and lumbar root syndromes.

- Is the pain confined to the back or does it radiate to the upper or lower limb?
- Is the pain exacerbated by coughing or sneezing?
- Did the pain begin suddenly or gradually?

OTHER CONDITIONS
Ankylosing spondylitis
In ankylosing spondylitis the patient, usually male, complains of spinal pain and stiffness, the latter improving with exercise.

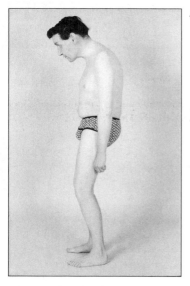

Advanced ankylosing spondylitis.

Rheumatoid arthritis
This complaint commonly involves the upper cervical spine.

Spinal tumours
Spinal tumours are usually metatastic from the prostate, breast, bronchus or kidney.

Tuberculosis
This disease most commonly involves the thoracic or lumbar spine.

TRAUMATIC LESIONS

Cervical spine injuries include atlanto-axial dislocation, fractures of the arch of the atlas and compression fractures of the vertebral bodies.

Thoracic and lumbar spine injuries include compression fractures and fractures of the transverse processes. Pathological fractures commonly occur at this level.

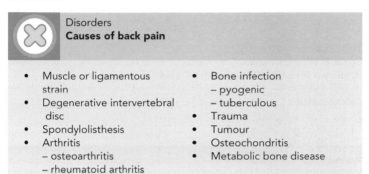

Disorders
Causes of back pain

- Muscle or ligamentous strain
- Degenerative intervertebral disc
- Spondylolisthesis
- Arthritis
  - osteoarthritis
  - rheumatoid arthritis
  - ankylosing spondylitis
- Bone infection
  - pyogenic
  - tuberculous
- Trauma
- Tumour
- Osteochondritis
- Metabolic bone disease

THE SHOULDER

INSPECTION AND PALPATION

Inspect the contour of the shoulder and its surrounding structures. Anterior dislocation results in a forward and downward displacement with alteration of the shoulder contour. Posterior dislocation is obvious.

JOINT MOVEMENT

Remember that most movement at the shoulder involves both the gleno-humeral joint and rotation of the scapula across the thorax.

Painful arc syndrome

The painful arc syndrome causes pain on shoulder elevation. Pain is absent initially, develops during abduction as elements of the cuff come into contact with the undersurface of the acromion, then disappears in the final part of abduction as the tendons fall away from the acromion.

Bicipital tendonitis

In bicipital tendonitis, tenosynovitis involves the long head of the biceps. The patient complains of pain in the anterior aspect of the shoulder and arm.

Traumatic lesions

Traumatic lesions include dislocation, fracture dislocation and fractures of the neck of the humerus.

MUSCLE FUNCTION

If shoulder movements are free and painless, the individual muscles concerned with movement around the joint can be tested.

Cervical radiculopathy

Cervical radiculopathy often affects the fifth nerve root. Weakness is found in the spinati, deltoid and biceps. The biceps and supinator reflexes are depressed.

Neuralgic amyotrophy

In neuralgic amyotrophy, severe pain around the shoulder is followed by patchy weakness and wasting in the shoulder girdle muscles.

Nerve palsies

Nerve palsies affecting the shoulder are rare.

THE ELBOW

INSPECTION AND PALPATION

Inspect the elbow joint from behind, comparing its alignment with the other arm. Palpate the subcutaneous border of the ulna, a common site for rheumatoid nodules, and then the lateral and medial epicondyles.

TRAUMATIC LESIONS

Include dislocations and fractures of the radial head and distal humerus. Dislocation is usually in a postero-lateral direction.

MUSCLE FUNCTION

Test the principal muscles concerned with elbow flexion and extension, together with pronation and supination.

A lesion of the C6 nerve root is common. Muscles that can be affected include the biceps, brachioradialis, supinator and triceps. In practice, triceps weakness predominates, with depression or loss of the triceps reflex. Any loss of sensation occupies the thumb and index finger.

THE FOREARM AND WRIST

INSPECTION AND PALPATION

Compare the size of the forearms, but remember that the dominant forearm tends to be rather larger. Compare the two wrists for size and for any evidence of swelling or deviation.

JOINT MOVEMENT

From the neutral position test flexion of the wrist (approximately 90°) then extension (approximately 70°). Now assess radial and ulnar deviation of the wrist. Wrist involvement is common in rheumatoid arthritis. Besides pain and limitation of movement, stretching of the ulnar collateral ligament allows the head of the ulna to subluxate upwards.

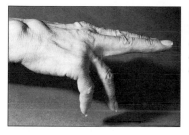

Elevation of the ulnar head in rheumatoid arthritis. The flexion deformity of the fourth and fifth digits is the result of rupture of their extensor tendons.

TRAUMATIC LESIONS

Fractures usually occur through the distal radius or ulnar, typically after a fall on an outstretched hand. Colles' fracture is sited about 1–2 cm above the distal end of the radius. The fracture is displaced dorsally. Smith's fracture is one at this site which is displaced in the opposite direction.

MUSCLE FUNCTION

Test the muscles acting at the wrist and the long flexors and extensors of the fingers.

A C7 root lesion affects the triceps together with wrist and finger extension. The triceps jerk may be depressed and sensory loss, if present, occurs over the middle finger.

A radial palsy most commonly results from damage to the nerve in the spinal groove. There is weakness of the supinator, brachioradialis and wrist and finger extension. The brachioradialis component of the supinator reflex is depressed.

Sensory loss is often slight, mainly involving an area of skin in the region of the anatomical snuff box.

THE HAND

A good way to examine the hands both for joint and muscle function is to ask the patient to sit opposite you with his hands spread on a flat surface.

Carefully palpate the joints. Is there joint tenderness? Assess the quality of any swelling.

In early rheumatoid arthritis, slight swelling of the proximal interphalangeal joints is accompanied by tenderness. At a later stage of the condition, substantial deformities occur accompanied by wasting of the small muscles.

Osteoarthritis commonly affects the carpometacarpal joint of the thumb in combination with changes in the distal interphalangeal joints.

Nodule formation on the flexor tendon can lead to the tendon being caught in a localised narrowing of the sheath. The result, trigger finger, is a flexion deformity from which the finger can be extended only by force.

TRAUMATIC LESIONS

Hand injuries include tendon damage and fractures. Severed extensor or flexor tendons require suturing to facilitate healing.

MOVEMENT

Test the range of movement in the thumb and fingers.

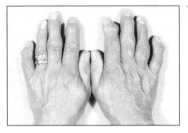

The square hand of osteoarthritis.

Questions to ask
Weakness of the hand

- Is the weakness associated with joint pain?
- Is the weakness confined to the muscles supplied by the median or ulnar nerve?
- If the weakness is global, are both hands or just one hand affected?
- Is there accompanying sensory loss?

THE HAND MUSCLES

INSPECTION

First inspect the dorsum of the hands. Wasting produces guttering between the extensor tendons, hollowing between the index finger and thumb, and loss of the convexity of the hypothenar eminence. Look for fasciculation. Now turn the hands over and inspect the palmar surfaces.

TESTING POWER

Start with a muscle supplied by the ulnar nerve. A good choice is the first dorsal interosseous. Now move on to muscles supplied by the median nerve. Start with abductor pollicis brevis then proceed to test opponens pollicis

CLINICAL APPLICATION

If the weakness is confined to the muscles of the thenar eminence, you are dealing with a distal median nerve lesion, most probably within the carpal tunnel. Weakness with or without wasting of the muscles of the thenar eminence is accompanied by a characteristic failure of the thumb to rotate during attempted opposition.

If the weakness is confined to the muscles supplied by the ulnar nerve, you next need to determine the site of the lesion. The most common site is in the region of the ulnar groove at the elbow, usually the consequence of recurrent trauma and angulation. The hand muscles affected include the interossei, the hypothenar muscles and the third and fourth lumbricals.

If there is weakness of all the small hand muscles, you are probably dealing with a proximal lesion. If the other hand is normal, suspect a problem at the level of the brachial plexus or T1 root. The cervical rib (thoracic outlet) syndrome results from compression of the C8 and T1 roots or the lower trunk of the plexus, by a fibrous band passing from the transverse process of the seventh cervical vertebra to the first rib. If you find bilateral weakness, with or without wasting, of the small hand muscles, you are dealing with a more diffuse process. You have to consider a peripheral neuropathy or a lesion of the anterior horn cell (e.g. syringomyelia or motor neuron disease).

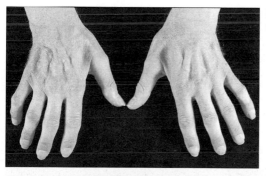

Bilateral ulnar nerve lesions.

THE HIP

INSPECTION AND PALPATION

Begin with the patient standing. Look for evidence of shortening of one of the legs. Compensation for this is achieved by a scoliotic posture or by flexion of the longer leg. An abduction deformity is compensated by flexion of the ipsilateral knee and adduction deformity by flexing the contralateral knee. A flexion deformity is compensated by an exaggerated lordosis.

With the patient still standing, assess the integrity of each hip joint and its surrounding muscles by asking the patient to stand first on one leg and then the other (Trendelenberg's test).

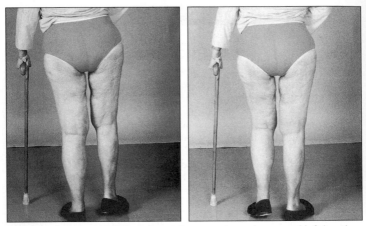

Trendelenberg's sign. When the patient stands on the normal left leg the pelvis tilts to the left (left). When she stands on the right leg (where there was osteoarthritis at the hip) the pelvis fails to tilt to the right (right).

> ### ✖ Disorders
> **Causes of hip pain**
>
> - Trauma
>   - dislocation
> - Arthritis
>   - osteoarthritis
>   - rheumatoid arthritis
> - Slipped femoral epiphysis
> - Osteochondritis (Perthe's disease)
> - Infection
>   - e.g. osteomyelitis

MEASUREMENT OF LIMB LENGTH

When measuring limb length, you need to distinguish between true and apparent shortening. Make sure that the position of the two hip joints is comparable when measuring. The true length is measured from the anterior superior iliac spine to the medial malleolus.

JOINT MOVEMENT

To test flexion, bend the leg, with the knee flexed, into the abdomen. Extension is best assessed by standing behind the patient and drawing the leg backwards until the point at which the pelvis starts to rotate. Abduction is measured by taking the leg outwards, again to the point where, by using the opposite hand, the pelvis is felt to move. Internal and external rotation are tested with the hip and knee flexed to 90°.

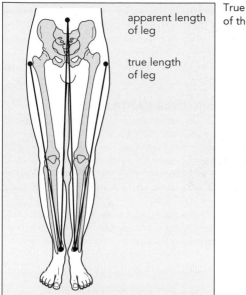

apparent length
of leg

true length
of leg

True and apparent lengths
of the lower limbs.

TRAUMATIC LESIONS

Dislocations are usually posterior and may then be accompanied by acetabular fractures. The leg is internally rotated, adducted and flexed. Fractures of the neck of the femur are commonplace in elderly people. The leg may be shortened and externally rotated. Fractures of the femoral shaft are either traumatic or pathological.

Muscle function

Test the power of hip flexion, extension, abduction and adduction. Sciatic palsies are associated with pelvic trauma, injuries to the buttock or thigh and infiltration by tumour.

THE KNEE

INSPECTION AND PALPATION

With the patient standing, look for a knee deformity, either genu valgum (knock-knee) or genu varum (bow leg). Next look for an effusion. If this is large, the swelling will extend from the suprapatellar region down either side of the patella. Smaller effusions are only detectable by palpation.

JOINT MOVEMENT

Test the range of movement with the patient lying supine.

STABILITY

To test the collateral ligaments, attempt to abduct and adduct the lower leg. If there is lateral instability, record its degree. For the assessment of cruciate ligaments, bend the knee to a slight angle, sit on the patient's foot then tense the lower leg first forwards then backwards. If either ligament is lax, excessive movement will occur.

ASSESSMENT OF THE SEMILUNAR CARTILAGES

In order to test the integrity of the semilunar cartilages, bend the hip and knee to 90° and grip the heel with your right hand while pressing on the medial then lateral cartilage with your left. Now internally and externally rotate the tibia while extending the knee. If there is a cartilage tear, its engagement between the tibia and femur during the manoeuvre leads to severe pain, a clunking noise and, sometimes, actual locking of the joint (McMurray's test).

In osteoarthritis, peri-articular tenderness, particularly at the insertion of the capsule and collateral ligaments, is an important diagnostic clue. Later, bony swellings around the joint and secondary quadriceps wasting are common.

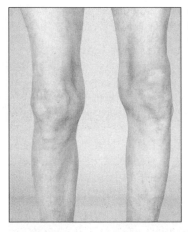

Osteoarthritis of the knee. Bony swellings associated with quadriceps wasting.

TRAUMATIC LESIONS

With ligament rupture, the consequent joint instability necessitates surgical repair. Meniscal tears tend to occur in young people as the consequence of a twisting injury. The medial meniscus is usually affected. Effusion appears and the knee may lock, inhibiting complete extension. The torn elements are removed arthroscopically.

Patella dislocation occurs laterally and tends to be recurrent. Total knee dislocation is unusual and generally the consequence of a road traffic accident.

MUSCLE FUNCTION

Test the muscles responsible for knee extension and flexion, the quadriceps and the hamstrings, respectively.

If the knee joint is normal, unilateral quadriceps weakness suggests either a femoral neuropathy or an L3 root syndrome. An obturator palsy can follow surgery or pelvic fracture or be secondary to obturator hernia. Weakness is confined to the thigh adductors with altered sensation over the thigh's inner aspect.

Meralgia paraesthetica

The patient with meralgia paraesthetica complains of pain, tingling and numbness over the anterolateral aspect of the thigh. There are no motor changes. The condition is caused by compression of the lateral cutaneous nerve of the thigh at the level of the groin.

Disorders
Causes of knee pain

- Trauma
  - fracture
  - dislocation
  - ligament damage
  - cartilage damage
- Arthitis
  - osteoarthritis
  - rheumatoid arthritis
- Osteochondritis dissecans
- Infection
  - e.g. osteomyelitis
- Bone tumours
- Referred
  - e.g. from the hip

THE ANKLE AND FOOT

INSPECTION AND PALPATION

To assess the alignment of the feet at the subtalar joints, look at the ankles from behind with the patient standing. In a varus deformity, the foot will be deviated towards the midline, in a valgus deformity away from it. Now palpate the margins of the ankle joint. In an inflammatory arthropathy, the whole joint is likely to be tender, with corresponding pain on all movement. Next palpate the heel and Achilles tendon. The latter is a fairly common site for rheumatoid nodules.

Deformity of the foot is common. In flat foot, the longitudinal arch is lost with the consequence that most or the whole of the sole comes into contact with the ground. In pes cavus, the arch of the foot is exaggerated with accompanying hyperextension of the toes. Hallux valgus predominates in women. It consists of abnormal adduction of the big toe at the metatarsophalangeal joint, with a bursa at the pressure point over the head of the first metatarsal. A hammer toe is characterised by hyperextension at the metatarsophalangeal joint with flexion at the interphalangeal joint.

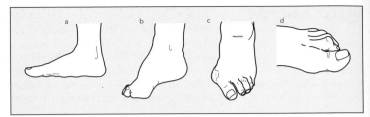

Foot deformities. (a) Pes planus, (b) pes cavus, (c) hallux valgus and (d) hammer toe.

- Has the deformity been present from birth?
- Does it affect both feet?
- Is it associated with joint pain or tenderness?

JOINT MOVEMENT

The ankle joint proper is concerned with plantar and dorsiflexion. Inversion and eversion of the foot occur both at the subtalar and midtarsal joints.

TRAUMATIC LESIONS

Pott's fracture is a fracture–dislocation of the ankle, sometimes requiring open reduction and fixation.

Rupture of the Achilles tendon results in pain in the heel. The calf is swollen with a palpable gap in the tendon. Open operation is called for if the condition is detected early.

Osteoarthritis can affect both the ankle and the foot.

Gout typically affects the same joint. In an acute attack, there is intense pain associated with swelling and erythema of the overlying skin.

Rheumatoid arthritis involves both the ankle and the foot. When the disease is established, subluxation of the metatarsophalangeal joint is associated with flexion deformity at the proximal interphalangeal joints.

MUSCLE FUNCTION

Test the individual muscles concerned with movement at the ankle and foot. Start with the plantar and dorsiflexors of the ankle, then of the toes. Specifically test the extensor of the big toe, extensor hallucis longus Finally, test the evertors and invertors of the foot.

Lumbar spondylosis commonly affects the L5 and S1 roots.

In lateral popliteal palsy, there is weakness of dorsiflexion of the foot and toes and of the foot everters. The sensory change is often relatively inconspicuous.

PATTERNS OF WEAKNESS IN MUSCLE DISEASE

Certain characteristics support a clinical diagnosis of primary muscle disease. The weakness, which is usually symmetrical, tends to predominate proximally. In the upper limbs, the periscapular muscles and deltoid are weak but the hand muscles are spared. In the lower limbs, weakness of hip flexion and extension is often conspicuous. The patient adopts a lordotic posture and has a waddling gait.

Trendelenberg's sign is likely to be positive bilaterally. There is particular difficulty getting upright from a lying position. Typically, the patient turns into the prone position, kneels then climbs up his or her legs using the upper limbs in order to extend the trunk (Gowers' manoeuvre). In some of the muscular dystrophies, pseudohypertrophy of muscle occurs because of infiltration by fat and connective tissue. Having completed the limb assessment of joint and muscle, examine the gait formally. If the patient has described a substantial problem with gait, be ready to provide support when the patient starts to walk. Observe both the pattern of leg movement and the posture of the arms together with control of the trunk. If gait appears normal, ask the patient to walk heel-toe, that is, 'as if on a tightrope'. If the patient appears nervous, walk alongside them.

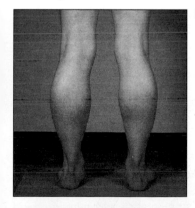

Pseudohypertrophy of the calves.

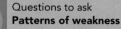

? Questions to ask
Patterns of weakness

- Is the weakness associated with sensory symptoms or signs?
- Is there a family history of muscle disease?
- Is the weakness symmetrical?
- Is the weakness predominantly proximal or distal?

SPASTIC GAIT
In a hemiplegia, the arm is held flexed and adducted while the leg is extended. In order to move the leg, the patient tilts the pelvis which produces an outward and forward loop of the leg (circumduction).

FOOT DROP GAIT
Foot drop can be either unilateral or bilateral. The former is usually the result of a lateral popliteal palsy, the latter the consequence of a peripheral neuropathy.

ATAXIC GAIT
An ataxic gait can reflect either loss of sensory information from the feet or a disorder of cerebellar function. In the former case, the patient stamps the feet down in order to overcome the instability.

Cerebellar disease leads to a broad-based gait that is unaffected by the presence or absence of visual information.

WADDLING GAIT
Patients with substantial proximal lower limb weakness waddle from side-to-side as they walk, from a failure to tilt the pelvis when one leg is raised from the ground.

PARKINSONIAN GAIT
Patients with Parkinson's disease develop an increasingly flexed posture. Stride length diminishes and one or both arms fail to swing.

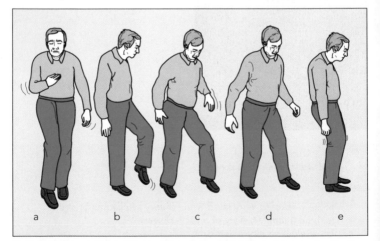

Gait disorders. (a) Hemiplegic, (b) unilateral foot drop, (c) sensory ataxia, (d) cerebellar ataxia and (e) Parkinsonism.

APRAXIC GAIT

In certain conditions (e.g. normal pressure hydrocephalus), there is a particular problem with the organisation of gait even though other skilled lower limb movements are spared.

HYSTERICAL GAIT

Falls and injuries do not exclude the possibility of a hysterical conversion reaction. There is often a violently positive Romberg's test which the patient self-corrects.

Examination of elderly people
Bones, muscles and joints

- Muscle strength declines with age. For example, grip strength falls by approximately 50% between the ages of 25 and 80 years.
- Muscle bulk declines with age. For example, in the small hand muscles.
- Some degree of ulnar deviation at the wrists can occur with ageing.
- The range of joing movement lessens with age.
- Gait becomes less certain in elderly people with a tendency for the steps to shorten.
- Elderly people tend to stand with slightly flexed hips and knees.

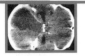

11. The Nervous System

SYMPTOMS

MOOD
This can be assessed by direct questioning but also by observation of the patient's behaviour.

MEMORY
The demented patient often denies loss of memory, particularly once the condition is established. In the early stages, however, patients can retain awareness of their difficulty, and sometimes volunteer that remote memory is partly spared.

SPEECH
Aphasic patients usually retain insight into their word-finding difficulty. Listening to the history allows estimation of the degree of fluency in speech production.

GEOGRAPHICAL ORIENTATION
The first sign of geographical disorientation may be the inability to follow a familiar route.

DRESSING
Ask the patient if they have encountered any problems while dressing.

EXAMINATION

ORIENTATION
Begin by assessing the patient's orientation in time and space. Establish the patient's age and ask the time, date and the name of the hospital in which the interview is taking place.

MEMORY
Immediate recall
For testing recall, use digit repetition, although a normal response also requires intact attention and adequate comprehension. The performance of serial sevens (subtracting seven serially from 100) is dependent on many factors. An abnormal response to this test does not specifically identify the patient with dementia.

Recent memory (new learning ability)
The examination begins by asking the patient about recent events. Next ask

the patient to memorise three objects or, alternatively, a name, an address and a flower. Over the next 10 min distract the patient so that there is no opportunity for mental rehearsal, then ask the patient to repeat the data.

Visual memory can be tested by displaying drawings for a 5-s period then asking the patient to reproduce the design 10 s later.

Remote memory
Ask the patient about schooling, childhood, work history, marriage and, if relevant, the ages of their children.

INTELLIGENCE
Testing a patient's knowledge and abstract thinking must be performed in the light of their social background.

Level of information
Ask the patient to give an account of recent events and their understanding of them.

Calculation
Give the patient simple addition, subtraction, multiplication and division sums.

Proverb interpretation
Interpretation of proverbs tests both general knowledge and capacity for abstract thinking.

Constructional ability
Constructional ability can be tested by asking the patient to copy designs of increasing complexity.

GEOGRAPHICAL ORIENTATION
Evidence concerning this may have been forthcoming during history taking but to test it specifically ask the patient to draw an outline of their native country placing within it a few of the principal cities.

SPEECH AND SPEECH DEFECTS
Determine the patient's handedness.

Dysarthria
This is a defect of articulation without any disturbance of language function.

Dysphonia
Dysphonia is a defect of speech volume and is usually the result of a disorder limiting the excursion either of the muscles of respiration or of the vocal cords.

Aphasia
This is a defect of language function in which there is either abnormal comprehension or production of speech or both. Aphasic speech lacks grammatical content, displays word-finding difficulty and contains word substitutions (paraphasias).

Fluency
Fluency may be defined as the amount of speech produced in a given period of time. Nonfluent speech, therefore, contains a limited number of words. Fluent dysphasia is near or even above normal in terms of output.

Comprehension
In testing comprehension, increasingly complex questions can be asked but all should be answerable by a simple yes or no response.

Repetition
Start by asking the patient to repeat simple words, then give sentences of increasing complexity.

Naming
A naming defect is found in virtually all dysphasic patients.

Reading
Reading assessment must take account of educational background.

Writing
Agraphia is an inevitable accompaniment of aphasia.

Praxis
Apraxia is a disorder of skilled movement not attributable to weakness, incoordination, sensory loss or a failure of comprehension. A defect for a single skilled task is termed ideomotor apraxia. Ideational apraxia is a failure to perform a more complex sequence of skilled activity.

Right–left orientation
A proportion of normal individuals have some problem with right–left orientation.

Agnosia
Patients with visual agnosia are unable to recognise objects they see, despite intact visual pathways and speech capacity.

Conclusion
Screening tests have been devised that allow a rapid assessment of function. Such tests, for example, the mini-mental state test are useful.

Orientation

1. What is the year, season, date, month, day? (One point for each correct answer.)
2. Where are we? Country, county, town, hospital, floor? (One point for each correct answer.)

Registration

3. Name three objects taking 1 s to say each. Then ask the patient to repeat them. One point for each correct answer. Repeat the questions until the patient learns all three.

Attention and calculation

4. Serial sevens. One point for each correct answer. Stop after five answers. Alternative, spell 'world' backwards.

Recall

5. Ask for the names of the three objects asked in Question 3. One point for each correct answer.

Language

6. Point to a pencil and a watch. Have the patient name them for you. One point for each correct answer.
7. Have the patient repeat 'No, ifs, ands or buts.' One point.
8. Have the patient follow a three-stage command: 'Take the paper in your right hand, fold the paper in half, put the paper on the floor.' Three points.
9. Have the patient read and obey the following: Close your eyes. (Write this in large letters.) One point.
10. Have the patient write a sentence of his or her own choice. (The sentence must contain a subject and an object and make some sense.) Ignore spelling errors when scoring. One point.
11. Have the patient draw two intersecting pentagons with equal sides. Give one point if all the sides and angles are preserved and if the intersecting sides form a quadrangle.

Maximum score = 30 points

The mini-mental state test.

PRIMITIVE REFLEXES

At this stage it is worth testing a number of primitive reflexes before passing on to the cranial nerve examination.

The glabellar tap

Tap repetitively with the tip of your index finger on the glabella. The blinking response should inhibit after three to four taps. In dementia and Parkinson's disease, the response persists.

The palmo-mental reflex

Apply firm and fairly sharp pressure to the palm of the hand alongside the thenar eminence. If the response is positive, contraction of the ipsilateral mentalis causes a puckering of the chin.

Pout and suckling reflexes

A positive pout response results in protrusion of the lips when they are lightly tapped by the index finger. A positive suckling reflex consists of a suckling movement of the lips when the angle of the mouth is stimulated.

Grasp reflex

Stroke firmly across the palmar surface of the hand from the radial to the ulnar aspect. In a positive response, the examiner's hand is gripped by the patient's fingers making release difficult. A foot grasp reflex is elicited by stroking the sole of the foot towards the toes with the handle of the patella hammer. A positive response leads to plantar flexion of the toes.

Disorders
Higher cortical function and speech

- **Dementia**
  – Alzheimer's disease
- **Amnesia**
  – postherpes simplex encephalitis
- **Dysarthria**
  – brainstem stroke
- **Dysphonia**
  – myasthenia gravis
- **Dysphasia**
  – Broca type, Wernicke type
- **Apraxia**
  – corpus callosum lesions
- **Grasp reflex**
  – frontal lobe tumours

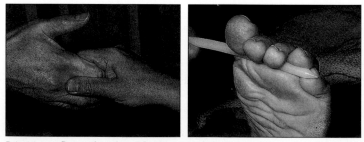

Primitive reflexes (hand and foot grasp).

CLINICAL APPLICATION

DEMENTIA
The majority of patients with dementia have Alzheimer's disease or senile dementia of Alzheimer-type. Most of the remainder have either cerebro-vascular disease or a mixed pathology.

AMNESIA
Damage to the limbic system results in a failure to learn new memories (ante-grade amnesia) associated with a defect of memory for the more recent past (retrograde amnesia).

DYSCALCULIA
Dyscalculia can occur with bilateral or unilateral lesions.

CONSTRUCTIONAL APRAXIA AND GEOGRAPHICAL DISORIENTATION
Constructional difficulty is particularly associated with parietal lobe lesions of the nondominant hemisphere.

DYSARTHRIA
Bulbar palsy
Combined weakness of the lips, tongue and palate.

Pseudobulbar palsy
Speech is hesitant and has an explosive, strangulated quality.

Vocal cord paralysis
With unilateral paresis, speech is hoarse and of reduced volume. With bi-lateral paresis speech is virtually lost.

Cerebellar lesions
There is loss of speech rhythm with fluctuation in volume and inflexion. Slurring and staccato elements are found.

DYSPHONIA
Many patients who lose their voice do not have organic disease. In spastic dysphonia, a form of dystonia, inappropriate muscle contraction produces strained and strangulated speech.

APHASIA
Nonfluent speech is associated with anterior hemisphere lesions and fluent speech with posterior hemisphere lesions.

Broca's aphasia
The output is nonfluent and usually dysarthric, Comprehension is intact except for complex phrases and there are naming errors.

Transcortical motor aphasia
This is similar to Broca's aphasia except that repetition is retained. The pathological process is located above or anterior to Broca's area.

Wernicke's aphasia
Here the patient has fluent, easily articulated speech but there are frequent paraphasias and meaning is largely absent. Comprehension and repetition are severely impaired.

Conduction aphasia
Conduction aphasia is fluent but not to the degree seen in Wernicke's aphasia. Interruptions to the speech rhythm are frequent but there is no dysarthria. Naming is imperfect but comprehension good. Despite this, repetition is severely abnormal.

Transcortical sensory aphasia
Transcortical sensory aphasia is fluent but frequently interrupted by repetition of words or phrases initiated by the examiner (echolalia). Despite the readiness and accuracy of the patient's repetition, comprehension is severely impaired.

Anomic aphasia
Anomic aphasia is fluent and interrupted more by pauses than by paraphasic substitutions. Anomic aphasia can be the final stage of recovery from other forms of aphasia.

Global aphasia
Global aphasia affects all aspects of speech function. Output is nonfluent and comprehension, repetition, naming, reading and writing are all affected, often to a severe degree.

DYSLEXIA AND ALEXIA
Dyslexia refers to developmental disorders of reading and alexia refers to disorders secondary to acquired brain damage.

AGRAPHIA
Although virtually all aphasic patients have agraphia, many patients with agraphia are not aphasic.

APRAXIA
The pathway involved in performing a skilled task to command begins in the auditory association cortex of the dominant hemisphere then passes to the

parietal association cortex, subsequently travelling forwards to the premotor cortex and finally the motor cortex itself. Interruption of this pathway at any point results in an ideomotor apraxia affecting both the dominant and non-dominant hands.

RIGHT–LEFT DISORIENTATION

Right–left disorientation is usually the result of a posteriorly placed dominant hemisphere lesion.

VISUAL AGNOSIA

One form of visual agnosia is caused by a disconnection between the visual cortex and the speech area. In the other form of visual agnosia, recognition of objects fails but their use can be demonstrated if the object is placed in the hand.

PRIMITIVE REFLEXES

The palmo-mental reflex is found bilaterally in some normal individuals but a unilateral palmo-mental reflex suggests a contralateral frontal lobe lesion. Snout and suckling reflexes are elicited in patients with diffuse bilateral hemisphere disease. Bilateral grasp reflexes are of limited localising value but a unilateral response is associated with pathology in the contralateral frontal lobe. A foot grasp or tonic plantar reflex can be one of the earliest signs of a frontal lobe lesion.

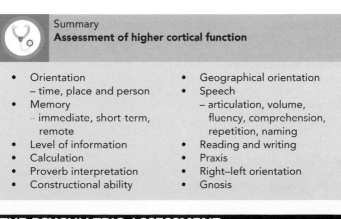

Summary
Assessment of higher cortical function

- Orientation
  – time, place and person
- Memory
  – immediate, short term, remote
- Level of information
- Calculation
- Proverb interpretation
- Constructional ability
- Geographical orientation
- Speech
  – articulation, volume, fluency, comprehension, repetition, naming
- Reading and writing
- Praxis
- Right–left orientation
- Gnosis

THE PSYCHIATRIC ASSESSMENT

SYMPTOMS

The most important part of the psychiatric assessment is the interview, in which the patient's mood and personality can be gauged while the history unfolds.

Anxiety
Patients will usually complain specifically of anxiety but sometimes its somatic manifestations, for example, palpitations, sweating and tremulousness predominate.

Depression
The somatic manifestations of depression are often as conspicuous as the mood change itself.

Euphoria
There is likely to be a pressurised, manic quality to the patient's conversation accompanied by physical restlessness.

Obsessiveness
The obsessive patient has become a victim to ritualistic thoughts or actions.

Delusions
Delusions are ideas that cannot be dismissed by the patient despite evidence indicating their falsity. Paranoid delusions contain a persecutory element.

Abnormal perceptions
Illusions are misinterpretations of an external reality. Hallucinations are experiences that have no objective equivalent to explain them.

Visual hallucinations
These may be unformed, for example an ill-defined pattern of lights, or formed, the patient then describing individuals or animals, often of a frightening aspect.

Auditory hallucinations
Auditory hallucinations are also either unformed or formed.

Déja and jamais vu
Déja and jamais vu refer, respectively, to an intense feeling of a relived experience and to a sensation of strangeness in familiar surroundings. Both can occur in everyday life but when pathological are usually epileptic in origin.

Questions to ask
Psychiatric assessment

- Do you feel unduly anxious or depressed?
- Do you repeat certain tasks over and over again?
- Do you feel people are against you?
- Have you heard or seen things that are not there?
- Do you ever lose the sense of yourself or your environment?

Depersonalisation and derealisation

In depersonalisation the patient feels a sense of bodily strangeness, amounting at times to a sense of being outside the body, watching it as an external witness. Derealisation results in a sense of loss of reality of the environment.

OTHER ASPECTS OF THE HISTORY
Family history
Personal history
Past illness
Drug history
Personality profile

EXAMINATION

The concept of the psychiatric examination needs to be interpreted broadly. A physical examination is necessary but the most telling diagnostic details will be revealed by an exploration of the patient's mental state, emerging as much from the history as from the answers to specific questions.

CLINICAL APPLICATION

ORGANIC MENTAL STATES
In organic mental states, a specific pathological basis for the mental disorder has been established. The principal chronic organic mental state is dementia.

FUNCTIONAL MENTAL STATES
In functional mental states, a specific underlying pathological or metabolic cause has not been identified. Psychotic states are those in which the individual has lost insight and neurotic states are those in which insight is preserved.

PHOBIAS
Phobias are a particular form of anxiety triggered by a specific environment or circumstance.

DEPRESSIVE ILLNESS
Depressive illnesses include those triggered primarily by genetic or constitutional factors (endogenous) and those precipitated by adverse external events (reactive).

MANIA AND HYPOMANIA
In mania and hypomania (its lesser form), there is pressure of talk and physical activity.

SCHIZOPHRENIA

Schizophrenia has been classified into a number of types, although the entities defined are not absolutely distinct. It is characterised by thought disorder, blunting of emotional responses, paranoid tendencies and perceptual disorders.

OBSESSIONAL STATES

In obsessional states, a preoccupation with mental or physical acts predominates.

HYSTERIA (CONVERSION HYSTERIA)

Hysteria is a disorder in which physical symptoms or signs exist for which there is no objective counterpart and which require, in the case of signs, an elaboration on the part of the patient of which he or she is unaware.

HYSTERICAL PERSONALITY

Hysterical personality is distinct from hysteria, although individuals with this personality trait may develop conversion reactions.

Questions to ask
Mental state

For anxiety
- Are the symptoms provoked by particular environments?

For depression
- Are there suicidal thoughts?

For schizophrenia
- Has the patient had auditory hallucinations?
- Does the patient believe his or her thoughts are controlled by others?

THE CRANIAL NERVES
THE OLFACTORY (FIRST) NERVE

Disorders
Disturbances of olfaction

- Post-traumatic anosmia
- Postinfective anosmia
- Olfactory hallucinations in complex partial seizures

EXAMINATION

The most convenient method for testing smell uses squeeze bottles bearing a nozzle that can be inserted into each nostril in turn. The patient is asked either to identify the smell or to describe its quality.

CLINICAL APPLICATION

Olfaction is commonly disturbed by upper respiratory tract infection or local nasal pathology. Smell sensitivity is diminished in dementia. Olfactory hallucinations occur in complex partial seizures (temporal lobe epilepsy).

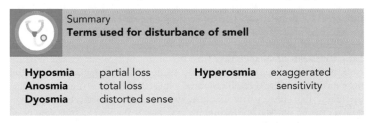

Summary
Terms used for disturbance of smell

Hyposmia	partial loss	**Hyperosmia**	exaggerated
Anosmia	total loss		sensitivity
Dyosmia	distorted sense		

THE OPTIC (SECOND) NERVE

A number of questions are appropriate when assessing the patient's complaint of vision loss or alteration.

Questions to ask
Visual disturbances

- Is the vision loss unilateral or bilateral?
- Is it confined to one area of the visual field?
- Are there positive as well as negative visual phenomena?
- Do colours appear different?

EXAMINATION

VISUAL ACUITY
The Snellen chart is used for testing distance vision.

Seat or stand the patient 6 m from the card. An acuity of 6/18, therefore, indicates that, at 6 m from the chart, the patient is able to read down only to the 18 m line. A visual acuity of less than 1/60 can be recorded as counting fingers, hand movements, perception of light or no perception of light. Near vision is tested using reading test types.

COLOUR VISION

Bedside tests of colour vision are designed principally to detect congenital defects.

VISUAL FIELDS

The field of vision to a coloured object, reflecting cone function, is more restricted than the field of a white object of the same size. Only the central portions of the two visual fields are binocular, the temporal margins being monocular.

For bedside testing of the visual field sit approximatley 1 m from the patient. For co-operative adults and older children, either finger movements or coloured objects can be used. If individual half fields are full, then the target object, usually your moving fingers, should be presented in both peripheral fields simultaneously.

Hand or finger movements are too crude a stimulus for assessing central field defects and here a small coloured object is used. It is useful to outline the blind spot first, partly because its successful identification increases confidence in one's own technique and partly because it indicates good fixation on the part of the patient.

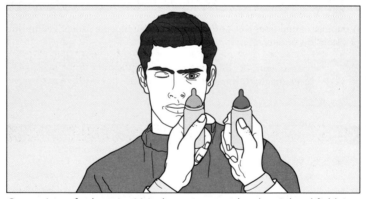

Comparison of colour sensitivity between central and peripheral field. In this patient with a central scotoma, the object appears lighter in the central field.

FUNDOSCOPY

Ask the patient to fixate on a distant target. If the patient wears glasses with a substantial correction, it sometimes facilitates the examination to perform it with the patient's glasses in place.

The optic disc is examined first to assess its shape, colour and clarity. The vessels are examined next. The arteries are narrower than the veins and a brighter colour. The retinal veins should be closely inspected where they enter the optic disc. In approximately 80% of normal individuals the veins pulsate. This pulsation ceases when cerebrospinal fluid (CSF) pressure exceeds 200 mm of water. The fundus is examined for the presence of haemorrhages and exudates, the positions of which are best shown by a small diagram in the patient's notes, or by a description that uses the optic disc as a clock face for localisation purposes, for example, 'one large haemorrhage at 6 o'clock, one disc diameter from the disc'.

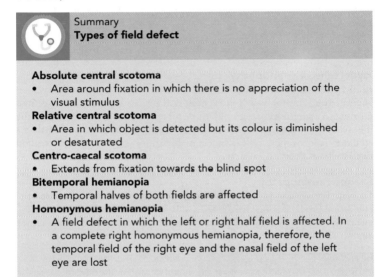

Summary
Types of field defect

Absolute central scotoma
- Area around fixation in which there is no appreciation of the visual stimulus

Relative central scotoma
- Area in which object is detected but its colour is diminished or desaturated

Centro-caecal scotoma
- Extends from fixation towards the blind spot

Bitemporal hemianopia
- Temporal halves of both fields are affected

Homonymous hemianopia
- A field defect in which the left or right half field is affected. In a complete right homonymous hemianopia, therefore, the temporal field of the right eye and the nasal field of the left eye are lost

CLINICAL APPLICATION

OPTIC ATROPHY

Optic atrophy follows any process that damages the ganglion cells or the axons between the retinal nerve fibre layer and the lateral geniculate body.

PAPILLOEDEMA

Patients with papilloedema often have no visual complaints, although some describe transient obscurations of vision either occurring spontaneously or triggered by postural change.

As papilloedema develops, swelling of the nerve fibre layer appears (best seen with a red-free light) within which haemorrhages are visible. The disc becomes hyperaemic (as a result of capillary dilatation) with a loss of definition of its margins and retinal venous pulsation disappears. In fully developed papilloedema there is engorgement of retinal veins, obscuration of the disc margin, flame haemorrhages and cotton wool spots (the consequence of retinal infarction). The vessels are tortuous. Often the only visual field change at this stage is an enlargement of the blind spot. In the later stages of papilloedema, hard exudates appear on the disc, which becomes atrophic and other visual field abnormalities appear, including arcuate fibre defects and peripheral constriction.

RETINAL VASCULAR DISEASE
Retinal artery and vein occlusion
After occlusion of the central retinal artery, the retina becomes pale and opaque with a cherry red spot at the macula. The optic disc, initially swollen, becomes atrophic. In central retinal vein occlusion there is swelling of the optic disc, dilatation of the retinal veins and fundal haemorrhages.

Hypertensive retinopathy
In hypertensive retinopathy, the light reflex from the arteriolar wall is abnormal and constriction of the venous wall appears at sites of arteriovenous crossing. A more reliable sign of hypertensive retinopathy is variation in the calibre of the retinal arterioles. As the retinopathy advances, haemorrhages and cotton wool spots appear and in malignant or accelerated hypertension disc swelling occurs.

Diabetic retinopathy
Diabetic retinopathy in its early stages principally affects the retinal micro-circulation producing the characteristic, although not pathognomonic, micro-aneurysm. Subsequently small haemorrhages, exudates and cotton wool spots appear.

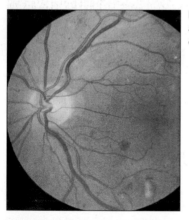

Diabetic retinopathy. Micro-aneurysms, haemorrhages, exudates and cotton wool spots.

GLAUCOMA
Glaucoma, characterised by raised intra-ocular pressure, can occur either secondarily to various ocular pathologies (e.g. uveitis) or in a primary form.

OPTIC NERVE DISEASE

In lesions of the optic nerve, the visual defect is monocular. Visual acuity is usually reduced and colour perception is disturbed. There is an afferent pupillary defect. The most likely visual field defect is a central scotoma.

CHIASMATIC LESIONS

Most chiasmatic syndromes are the result of compression by pituitary tumour, meningioma or craniopharyngioma. The result is a bitemporal hemianopia, although the type of defect relates to the position of the growth and its relation to the chiasm.

OPTIC TRACT AND LATERAL GENICULATE BODY LESIONS

These are uncommon. A lesion in the anterior part of the optic tract, before the homonymous fibres have joined, produces an incongruous homonymous hemianopia.

OPTIC RADIATION AND OCCIPITAL CORTEX LESIONS

The type of visual field loss from lesions of the optic radiation depends on their localisation. All the defects are homonymous but not necessarily congruous. Occipital lobe pathology produces congruous defects that can be total, quadrantic or scotomatous. An isolated homonymous hemianopia is usually occipital in origin and almost always due to vascular disease.

THE OCULOMOTOR, TROCHLEAR AND ABDUCENS (THIRD, FOURTH AND SIXTH) NERVES

SYMPTOMS

If the patient complains of ptosis, find out whether the problem is bilateral or unilateral and whether it fluctuates. For diplopia, a number of questions may help to suggest the underlying mechanism.

Questions to ask
Diplopia

- Is the diplopia relieved by covering one or other eye?
- Is the diplopia horizontal, vertical or oblique?
- Does the diplopia increase in one particular direction of gaze?
- Does the diplopia fluctuate or is it constant?

EXAMINATION

INSPECTION OF THE EYELIDS AND PUPILS

Note the position of the eyelids. If there is a ptosis, assess its fatiguability by asking the patient to sustain upward gaze. Next examine the pupils, which normally are circular and symmetrical, although a slight difference in size (anisocoria) of up to 2 mm is seen in some 20% of the population.

Pupillary light response

Now examine the pupillary light response using a bright pencil torch. The background illumination should be low and to prevent a near reaction the patient should fixate on a distant object. A defect of the afferent pupillary pathway is best appreciated by swinging the torch from one eye to the other.

Near reaction

If the light response is normal there is little point in testing the near reaction. If the light response is depressed, test the near reaction by asking the patient to fixate on a target (e.g. your forefinger) as it approaches the eyes.

INSPECTION OF EYE MOVEMENTS
Conjugate eye movements

Next assess conjugate eye movements. To test pursuit, ask the patient to follow a slowly moving target, first in the horizontal then in the vertical plane. If pursuit movements are slowed, brief saccades must be superimposed to allow the eyes to catch their target. To assess saccadic movements, ask the patient to rapidly fixate between two targets, for example, two fingers in the same plane.

Doll's head manoeuvre (oculocephalic reflex)

If the eyes fail to respond to a saccadic or pursuit stimulus, perform the doll's head manoeuvre. Ask the patient to fixate on your eyes, grasp the head and rotate it, first in the horizontal then in the vertical plane. An intact response (a measure of vestibular eye function) allows the patient's eyes to remain fixed on your own.

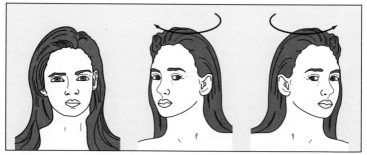

Performing the doll's head manoeuvre in the horizontal plane.

TESTING THE ACTION OF INDIVIDUAL EYE MUSCLES

In a strabismus, or squint, the axes of the eyes are no longer parallel. The strabismus is concomitant if the angle of deviation remains constant throughout the range of eye movement and incomitant if the angle of deviation varies. In the presence of a concomitant squint, covering the ixating eye produces a movement in the squinting eye that allows it to take up fixation. Most patients with concomitant squint do not complain of diplopia, a symptom that suggests a disorder of one or more of the extra-ocular muscles or their nerve supply.

Having confirmed that the diplopia is binocular (in other words, that it disappears when one or other eye is covered) ask the patient to look in the six directions illustrated in the figure below. The false image (which often appears indistinct or blurred) is peripheral to the true image and belongs to the affected eye. Having elicited the diplopia, cover first one eye, then the other, to establish to which eye the false image belongs. Observe if the patient has an abnormal head tilt as a compensation for the diplopia.

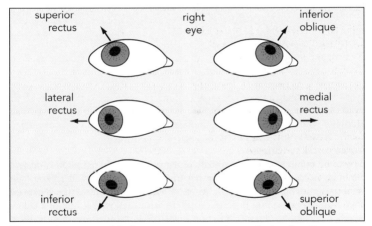

The muscles responsible for eye movements in particular directions.

Nystagmus

Note the presence of nystagmus and whether it is pendular or jerk. Record the amplitude (fine, medium or coarse), persistence and the direction of gaze in which it occurs. Additionally, indicate whether the movement is horizontal, vertical, rotary or a mixture of several types. First degree nystagmus to the left is a fast beating nystagmus to the left on left lateral gaze. In second and third degree nystagmus to the left, the same nystagmus is present on forward and right lateral gaze, respectively.

Optokinetic nystagmus

Optokinetic responses are assessed using a drum painted with vertical lines, which is rotated first in the horizontal and then in the vertical plane. As the patient looks at the drum a pursuit movement is seen in the direction of its rotation, followed by a saccade returning the eyes to the midposition.

CLINICAL APPLICATION

THE PUPIL
Horner's syndrome

Horner's syndrome results from interruption of the sympathetic fibres to the eye. The pupil is miosed and the palpebral fissure is narrowed because of mild ptosis of the upper lid and elevation of the lower lid. Although enophthalmos is suggested by the appearance of the eye, this is not confirmed by formal measurement. The distribution of sweating loss on the ipsilateral face depends on the site of the lesion. If there is uncertainty regarding the diagnosis, instill 4% cocaine into each eye. The normal pupil dilates, the affected pupil fails to do so, irrespective of the site of the lesion.

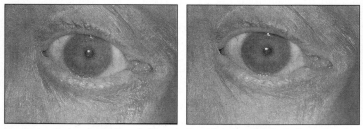

Horner's syndrome. Before (left) and after (right) instillation of cocaine.

Tonic pupil syndrome

The tonic pupil syndrome is usually unilateral. The affected pupil is dilated, although in long-standing cases it becomes progressively smaller. The light response is absent or markedly depressed and, consequently, in a darkened room, the affected pupil becomes smaller than its fellow because of a failure of reflex dilatation. The near reaction is delayed but sometimes more marked than that of the normal pupil. On relaxing the near effort, dilatation is delayed so that for a period the previously larger pupil is the smaller one. Tonic pupil syndrome is sometimes associated with depression of the deep tendon reflexes (Holmes–Adie syndrome).

Argyll Robertson pupil

The Argyll Robertson pupil is miosed, with a light response that is diminished compared with the near reaction (light–near dissociation). The pupil is often irregular with evidence of iris atrophy. When complete, the syndrome is pathognomonic of neurosyphilis.

Relative afferent pupillary defect

This results from a lesion of the afferent light reflex pathway between the retina and the optic tract. It is not found with disease of the lens or vitreous. In the presence of a unilateral optic nerve lesion, for example, caused by optic neuritis, the affected pupil dilates as the torch is swung onto it from the sound eye.

DISORDERS OF EYE MOVEMENTS
Gaze paresis
In an acute frontal lobe lesion, contralateral saccadic eye movements in the horizontal plane are depressed or absent and there is limb paresis ipsilateral to the gaze palsy. Both pursuit movements and the oculocephalic responses are spared. Saccades return later but now initiated by the contralateral frontal lobe. A lesion at the level of the paramedian pontine reticular formation produces an ipsilateral gaze paresis for both saccadic and pursuit movement. An ipsilateral pursuit paresis occurs with posterior hemisphere disease and is associated with a contralateral homonymous field defect.

A paresis of upward saccades, initially with relative preservation of pursuit, is a feature of the dorsal–midbrain (Parinaud's) syndrome. Other findings include impaired convergence and dilated, light–near dissociated pupils.

OTHER SACCADIC AND PURSUIT MOVEMENT DISORDERS
Saccadic slowing, accompanied by disorganised pursuit movements, is found in both Huntington's and Parkinson's disease. In progressive supranuclear palsy, downward saccades and pursuit fail first, followed by involvement of upward and, finally, horizontal movements. Doll's head movements are spared.

INTERNUCLEAR OPHTHALMOPLEGIA
A lesion of the medial longitudinal fasciculus leads to slowing, or total failure of medial rectus contraction during lateral gaze. There is usually an accompanying nystagmus in the abducting eye. Bilateral internuclear ophthalmoplegia is accompanied by upbeat vertical nystagmus.

THE 'ONE-AND-A-HALF' SYNDROME
If the lesion responsible for a unilateral internuclear ophthalmoplegia spreads into the pontine gaze centre, a more profound loss of ocular motility results. The only normal horizontal movement possible is abduction of the opposite eye.

Disorders
The pupil and eye movements

Pupillary syndromes
- Horner's
- Tonic pupil
- Argyll Robertson pupil
- Relative afferent pupillary defect

Eye movement disorders
- Gaze paresis
- Internuclear ophthalmoplegia

- One-and-a-half syndrome
- Abducens, trochlear and oculomotor nerve palsies

Nystagmus
- Congenital
- Vestibular
- Gaze-evoked
- Downbeat
- Convergence-retractory

ABDUCENS PALSY

A lesion of the sixth nerve nucleus produces a gaze paresis rather than an isolated lateral rectus weakness. The latter is usually due to a lesion of the central or peripheral course of the sixth nerve. The eye fails to abduct.

TROCHLEAR PALSY

Although normally a result of trochlear nerve palsy, weakness of the superior oblique muscle can occur with myasthenia or dysthyroid eye disease. The head tilts to the side opposite the affected eye and the patient complains of diplopia, particularly on downward gaze. There is defective depression of the adducted eye.

OCULOMOTOR PALSY

Nuclear oculomotor palsies tend to be either incomplete or complete but with pupillary sparing. A complete third nerve palsy cannot be nuclear unless there is involvement of the contralateral superior rectus muscle. Peripheral third nerve lesions are commonly caused by diabetes. The paresis is typically painful and pupil-sparing in about 50% of patients. In a complete third nerve palsy there is a substantial ptosis and the eye is deviated laterally and slightly downwards. Compression of the oculomotor nerve, for example, by a posterior communicating aneurysm, almost always results in pupillary dilatation.

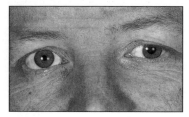

Left third nerve paresis. The pupil is dilated.

COMBINED PALSIES

A lesion within the cavernous sinus, for example, a cavernous aneurysm, is liable to affect the eye nerves in combination rather than individually. At risk are the third, fourth and sixth nerves, the first and second divisions of the trigeminal nerve and the ocular sympathetic fibres. A complex, mixed ophthalmoplegia without pupillary involvement, raises the possibility of myasthenia or dysthyroid eye disease.

NYSTAGMUS

Pendular – Usually congenital but sometimes found in brainstem vascular disease or multiple sclerosis.

Vestibular – If peripheral, usually both horizontal and rotary components and is suppressed by visual fixation. If central, more variable and unaffected by fixation.

Gaze-evoked – Often drug-induced but also seen with disease of the cerebellum or brainstem. Vertical components indicate brainstem or cerebellar disease.

Down-beat – When present on down and out gaze, very suggestive of a lesion at the foramen magnum, for example, Chiari malformation.

Convergence-retractory – Occurs in the dorsal-midbrain syndrome. Attempts at upwards saccades produce retractory movements of the globes.

End-point – Physiological. Occurs at extremes of lateral gaze and can affect one eye more than the other.

THE TRIGEMINAL (FIFTH) NERVE EXAMINATION

With the patient's eyes closed, test light touch by touching the appropriate areas of the face with a wisp of cotton wool. Now test pin prick sensation at the same sites. If there is a sensory loss confined to the trigeminal nerve distribution, the response to this stimulus becomes normal at the level of the vertex but well above the angle of the jaw.

THE CORNEAL RESPONSE

The corneal response is elicited by lightly touching the cornea with cotton wool. The patient's subjective reaction is assessed and the ipsilateral and contralateral blink reaction noted.

MOTOR

Look for muscle wasting before testing the muscles of mastication. Wasting of temporalis produces hollowing above the zygoma. The power of pterygoids and of masseter and temporalis can be assessed by resisting the patient's attempts at opening and closing the jaw respectively. In a unilateral trigeminal lesion, the jaw deviates to the paralysed side.

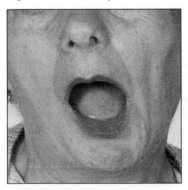

Left trigeminal nerve lesion. Jaw deviation to the left.

THE JAW JERK

Ask the patient to open the mouth slightly. Rest your index finger on the apex of the jaw and tap it with the patella hammer. The response, a contraction of the pterygoid muscles, varies widely in normal individuals.

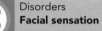

Disorders
Facial sensation

- Malignant invasion of the trigeminal nerve
- Isolated trigeminal neuropathy
- Involvement in the lateral medullary syndrome
- Involvement with cerebello-pontine angle tumours
- Sensory involvement with thalamic, capsular or cortical infarction

CLINICAL APPLICATION

MOTOR INVOLVEMENT

In a bilateral upper motor neuron syndrome, the jaw jerk is exaggerated.

SENSORY INVOLVEMENT

Malignant invasion of the nerve or its ganglion results in both sensory and motor deficit. In isolated trigeminal neuropathy, motor function is spared but there is progressive loss of facial sensation. In spinal lesions above C2, selective loss of facial pain and temperature sense is possible, sometimes with an 'onion ring' distribution. Loss of facial pain and temperature sense occurs ipsilaterally in the lateral medullary syndrome.

ALTERED CORNEAL RESPONSE

Loss of the corneal response may be the first or an early sign of trigeminal compression.

THE FACIAL (SEVENTH) NERVE

Questions to ask
Facial weakness of lower motor neuron type

- Have you noticed any loss of taste on the front part of the tongue?
- Have you noticed that noises appear excessively loud in the ear on the same side?
- Does the eye on that side still water?

SYMPTOMS

In a patient with a lower motor neuron facial weakness, certain questions may help to define the site of the lesion.

EXAMINATION

An asymmetry of blinking is a useful indicator of mild weakness of orbicularis oculi. Note any difference in the position of the two angles of the mouth but remember that in a long-standing facial weakness, fibrotic contracture of the muscles can elevate the angle of the mouth, suggesting that the facial weakness is on the other side. Bilateral facial weakness is easily overlooked. The face lacks expression and appears to sag.

Ask the patient to elevate the eyebrows then close the eyes tightly. Try to open the eyes by pressing the eyelids apart with your thumbs. Now ask the patient to blow out the cheeks, then purse the lips tightly together. Finally, ask the patient to tighten the neck muscles in order to assess platysma. Taste is difficult to test. For assessing seventh nerve function, the stimulus should be confined to the anterior two-thirds of the tongue, each side of which is tested separately. Sweet (sugar), salt, bitter (quinine) and sour (vinegar) solutions are applied in turn, the mouth being washed out with distilled water between testing.

CLINICAL APPLICATION

Upper motor neuron facial weakness

There is minimal asymmetry of frontalis contraction on the two sides but substantial asymmetry of the lower face.

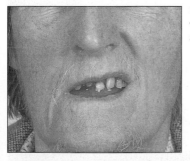

Upper motor neuron facial weakness. The patient has been asked to bare her teeth.

Lower motor neuron facial weakness

In a lower motor neuron facial weakness, all the facial muscles are equally affected unless the lesion lies so distally that it involves individual branches of the nerve. Involvement of the nerve immediately proximal to the origin of chorda tympani will result in loss of taste over the anterior two-thirds of the tongue; involvement proximal to the departure of the nerve to stapedius will result in hyperacusis. Loss of lacrimation is added to these other symptoms if the nerve is damaged at or proximal to the Gasserian ganglion.

Bell's palsy
Bell's palsy is an idiopathic paralysis of the facial nerve. If denervation occurs, regrowth of fibres may extend to muscles not originally part of their innervation (aberrant re-innervation).

Ramsay Hunt syndrome
The Ramsay Hunt syndrome is the consequence of herpetic involvement of the geniculate ganglion. A vesicular eruption can occur at a number of sites, including the pinna.

Facial movement disorders
Fasciculation – Virtually confined to patients with motor neuron disease.

Myokymia – Produces a fine, more or less continuous, shimmering contraction of some or all of the muscles supplied by the facial nerve.

Hemifacial spasm – Involuntary, haphazard contraction of facial muscle, often initially confined to orbicularis oculi. Eventually a mild facial weakness appears.

Blepharospasm – Forced involuntary repetitive blinking.

Tics – Stereotyped repetitive movements, at least in part under voluntary control.

Orofacial dyskinesia – Involuntary semi-repetitive contraction of muscles round the mouth, often with abnormal movements of the tongue.

THE ACOUSTIC (EIGHTH) NERVE

SYMPTOMS
Deafness
If the patient complains of deafness, determine the mode of onset, whether progressive or static, and whether unilateral or bilateral.

Vertigo
If the patient has vertigo, ascertain whether symptoms can be induced by certain postures or movements

EXAMINATION

AUDITORY FUNCTION
Each ear is tested separately. Ask the patient to occlude the ear not being tested by pressing on the tragus. Hearing sensitivity can be assessed by the

> **?** Questions to ask
> **Dizziness**
>
> - Does the patient describe dizziness or giddiness or is there an experience of rotation, either of the patient or of the environment (vertigo)?
> - Is the dizziness accompanied by an unsteadiness when walking?
> - Is any vertigo triggered only by a certain movement or head posture?

capacity to hear a whispered sound (normally possible at least 0.8 m away), a wristwatch (possible at approximately 0.75 m) or the sound of the fingers being rubbed together.

Rinne's test

Place a 512 Hz tuning fork on the mastoid process then hold it adjacent to the pinna. Normally, air conduction is better perceived than bone conduction (Rinne positive). In perceptive deafness, this discrepancy remains but in conductive deafness it is reversed.

Weber's test

Place a 512 Hz tuning fork at the midline over the vertex or on the forehead and ask the patient whether the sound appears equally loud in each ear or more so in one than the other. Normally, the sound is perceived equally by the two ears but it is heard better by the intact ear in perceptive deafness and by the affected ear in conductive deafness.

VESTIBULAR FUNCTION

If a patient complains of positional vertigo, then the effect of posture should be included in the examination. Position the patient at the edge of the examination couch, facing away from the edge, then depress the head and trunk so that the head is almost 30° below the horizontal but turned first to one side then the other. If nystagmus appears, record whether it begins immediately or after an interval, whether it persists or fatigues and if it then reappears when the patient returns to the sitting position.

CLINICAL APPLICATION

DEAFNESS

Conductive deafness is usually caused by either debris or wax in the external auditory meatus, loss of elasticity of the ossicular chain (otosclerosis) or disease of the middle ear. Nerve deafness occurs with end-organ change (e.g.

in Ménière's disease) or consequent to a disturbance of the auditory nerve itself (e.g. after occlusion of the internal auditory artery).

TINNITUS
Patients with tinnitus complain of noise in one or both ears. The symptom occurs with cochlear disease or damage, or with compression of the auditory nerve.

VERTIGO
Vertigo is a sense of rotation either of the individual or of the environment. Patients rarely complain of persistent vertigo, although many describe a persistent dizziness or giddiness, much less clear-cut symptoms that commonly elude diagnosis. Vertigo is usually a result of disruption of either the labyrinthine system (peripheral vertigo) or the central connections of the vestibular nerve (central vertigo).

Epidemic labyrinthitis and acute vestibular neuronitis
These diagnoses have been applied to patients who give a history of acute vertigo, often with vomiting, together with ataxia and malaise.

Benign positional vertigo
Benign positional vertigo is a more specific, peripheral, vestibular dysfunction. Patients complain of attacks of vertigo, typically triggered by lying down in bed on one particular side. Tests for positional nystagmus are positive.

Ménière's disease
In Ménière's disease, thought to be the consequence of a distension of the endolymphatic space, paroxysms of vertigo occur together with a persistent unilateral tinnitus and progressive sensorineural deafness.

Central vertigo
Central vertigo is likely to persist longer than peripheral vertigo and if posture related, is less likely to be delayed in onset or to fatigue after posture change than benign positional vertigo.

Disorders
Deafness and vertigo

Conductive deafness
- Wax
- Otosclerosis
- Middle ear disease

Perceptive deafness
- Ménière's disease
- Vascular event

- Acoustic neurinoma

Peripheral vertigo
- Vestibular neuronitis
- Benign positional vertigo
- Ménière's disease

Central vertigo
- Cerebrovascular disease

EXAMINATION OF THE GLOSSOPHARYNGEAL (NINTH) NERVE

Testing the gag reflex is an uncomfortable experience and should be performed only if there is a suspicion of a disturbance of the lower cranial nerves. Press the end of an orange stick first into one tonsillar fossa then the other. Besides confirming that the palate rises in the midline, ask the patient if the sensation is comparable on the two sides. In the presence of a glossopharyngeal lesion, the gag reflex is depressed or absent on that side.

CLINICAL APPLICATION

A destructive process in the region of the jugular foramen, most commonly a nasopharyngeal carcinoma, disrupts the ninth, tenth and eleventh cranial nerves. In the Chiari malformation, stretching of the ninth nerve can lead to depression of the gag reflex on one or both sides. Glossopharyngeal neuralgia usually results from distortion of the nerve by a tumour or a vascular anomaly. Paroxysms of pain in the tongue, soft palate or tonsil are triggered by swallowing, chewing or protruding the tongue.

EXAMINATION OF THE VAGUS (TENTH) NERVE

Bedside evaluation is confined to assessment of spontaneous and reflex movements of the uvula and posterior pharyngeal wall. A unilateral lesion of the vagus produces paralysis of the ipsilateral soft palate. At rest, the palate lies slightly lower on the affected side then deviates to the intact side during phonation or on testing the gag reflex. Bilateral palsies of the vagus produce severe palatal palsy, with nasal regurgitation and aphonia.

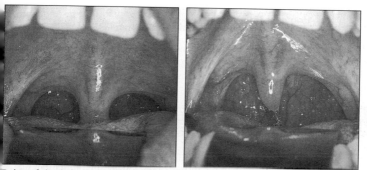

Palsy of the left vagus. The palate deviates to the right on phonation (right).

CLINICAL APPLICATION

Nuclear vagal lesions occur in polio and after lateral medullary infarction. Recurrent laryngeal palsies are usually left sided because of the longer course of the nerve on that side. Causes include aortic aneurysm, thyroid surgery and malignant invasion of the mediastinum.

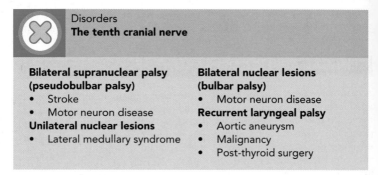

Disorders
The tenth cranial nerve

Bilateral supranuclear palsy (pseudobulbar palsy)
- Stroke
- Motor neuron disease

Unilateral nuclear lesions
- Lateral medullary syndrome

Bilateral nuclear lesions (bulbar palsy)
- Motor neuron disease

Recurrent laryngeal palsy
- Aortic aneurysm
- Malignancy
- Post-thyroid surgery

EXAMINATION OF THE ACCESSORY (ELEVENTH) NERVE

There is no way of assessing the innervation of the cranial component of the accessory nerve but that of the spinal component can be assessed by examining trapezius and sternomastoid. The function of trapezius is assessed by asking the patient to elevate the shoulder, first without, then with, resistance. The strength of contraction of sternomastoid can be gauged by asking the patient to rotate the head to the relevant side against resistance.

CLINICAL APPLICATION

In the presence of a hemiplegia, the trapezius muscle on the hemiplegic side is affected. A delay in shoulder shrug may be an early sign. Spasmodic torticollis is a focal dystonia particularly affecting the sternomastoid muscle.

EXAMINATION OF THE HYPOGLOSSAL (TWELFTH) NERVE

First inspect the tongue as it lies in the base of the oral cavity. Fasciculation imparts a shimmering motion to the surface of the tongue. Involuntary movements include a coarse tremor, for example, in Parkinson's disease and complex, unpredictable movements found in such conditions as Huntington's disease and orofacial dyskinesia. As the tongue wastes it becomes thinner and more wrinkled. Now ask the patient to protrude the tongue. Finally, ask the patient to move the tongue rapidly from side to side and assess its power by instructing the patient to push the tongue against the side of the cheek.

CLINICAL APPLICATION

UNILATERAL AND BILATERAL LOWER MOTOR NEURON LESIONS

In a unilateral hypoglossal nerve lesion, there is focal atrophy, fasciculation and deviation to the paralysed side. Bilateral involvement of the lower motor neuron projections to the tongue is usually part of a bulbar palsy. There is additional involvement of the other lower brainstem motor nuclei, resulting in dysphagia and dysarthria. The tongue is wasted and immobile.

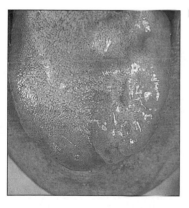

Left hypoglossal nerve lesion.

UNILATERAL UPPER MOTOR NEURON LESION

A unilateral upper motor neuron lesion has little effect on tongue function, although it may protrude slightly to the side of the hemiparesis.

BILATERAL UPPER MOTOR NEURON LESION

Bilateral involvement of the pyramidal projections to the brainstem nuclei, usually the consequence of cerebrovascular disease, results in a pseudobulbar palsy. There is dysphagia, dysarthria and emotional lability. The tongue is stiff and immobile and there is weakness of palatal elevation combined with a brisk gag reflex and jaw jerk.

> **Summary**
> **Cranial nerve examination**
>
> | | |
> |---|---|
> | I | Examine smell in each nostril |
> | II | Examine visual acuity, visual field, fundus and pupillary light response |
> | III, IV, VI | Examine eye movements and near reaction. Check for nystagmus |
> | V | Examine motor and sensory innervation plus the jaw jerk and the corneal response |
> | VII | Examine the muscles of facial expression (plus buccinator) and taste over the anterior two-thirds of the tongue |
> | VIII | Examine hearing and perform Rinne's and Weber's tests |
> | IX | Examine pain sensation in the tonsillar fossae |
> | X | Examine palatal movement plus the gag reflex |
> | XI | Examine sternomastoid and the upper fibres of the trapezius |
> | XII | Examine tongue movements and appearance |

THE MOTOR SYSTEM

The major supraspinal influences on motor activity are the sensorimotor cortex (exerting its role primarily through the pyramidal system), the basal ganglia, a number of tracts descending from the brainstem and the cerebellum. The upper motor neuron defines that part of the motor pathway between the cerebral cortex and the anterior horn cell. The lower motor neuron consists of the anterior horn cell and its motor axon.

SYMPTOMS

When recording a complaint of weakness, determine its mode of onset, its distribution, whether it fluctuates in severity and whether it is associated with feelings of stiffness in the affected part.

EXAMINATION

A detailed outline of the limb muscles and their examination is contained in Chapter 10. This section concentrates on an overview of patterns of weakness and how that pattern is helpful in diagnosis.

APPEARANCE

Some thinning of the small hand muscles is common in elderly people but is not associated with weakness. A global loss of muscle bulk is more likely to

? Questions to ask
Muscle weakness

- Is the weakness confined to one limb or to one side of the body?
- Is the weakness static, progressive or fluctuant?
- Is the weakness accompanied by a feeling of stiffness or is the affected limb floppy?

be the result of either impaired nutrition or malignancy rather than neurological disease. Focal muscle wasting can rapidly follow injury of a joint with consequent immobilization. The pattern of wasting often suggests a particular peripheral nerve or root disorder.

While inspecting the muscle, look for spontaneous contractions. Fasciculation is caused by spontaneous contraction of the fibres belonging to a single motor unit. Muscles may hypertrophy as well as atrophy. Pseudo-hypertrophic muscles are infiltrated by fat and connective tissue and are weak on formal testing

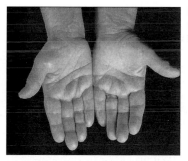

Focal wasting of the thenar eminence secondary to median nerve compression.

TONE
Ensure that the patient is comfortable and warm. First observe the limb posture, this may indicate the distribution of altered tone between the flexors and extensors of the limb. For screening purposes, assess flexion and extension at the elbow, pronation and supination of the forearm and flexion and extension at the knee, using a range of speeds rather than a fixed velocity. Remember to take account of any painful limb or joint.

Spastic limbs
In spastic limbs, at a critical velocity a catch appears that is absent during slower displacements. Subsequently, the hypertonus fades away as stretch continues. In the upper limbs it predominates in flexors and is more evident when the forearm is supinated than when it is pronated. In the lower limb it is greater in quadriceps than in the hamstrings.

Rigidity

Rigidity is more uniformly distributed in the limb. It may begin unilaterally and is sometimes easier to detect in one joint rather than another. The resistance is felt at low speeds of displacement and does not 'melt away'. If you have doubts regarding an increase in tone, ask the patient either to clench their teeth or grip the hand not being tested. In patients with rigidity, the increased tone becomes more evident during this procedure. At times rigidity is not uniform but fluctuates in a phasic manner, aptly described as cogwheeling.

Gegenhalten

A more diffuse increase in tone, Gegenhalten, can be found in patients with an altered level of consciousness and in individuals with frontal lobe lesions.

Hypotonia

The limb is floppy and is liable to show abnormal excursions when moved passively. Hypotonia occurs in the presence of a lower motor neuron lesion and in cerebellar disease.

Summary
Definitions of paralysis

Paresis	Partial paralysis
Plegia	Complete paralysis
Monoplegia	Involvement of a single limb
Hemiplegia	Involvement of one-half of the body
Paraplegia	Paralysis of the legs
Tetraplegia	Paralysis of all four limbs

MUSCLE POWER

The UK Medical Research Council system of classification is recommended for grading muscle weakness. In practice, grades 4 and 5 are separated by a wide range of strength but as you gain experience you can overcome this problem by using the grades 4+, 4++ and 5-.

In the upper limbs, first ask the patient to shrug his or her shoulders. In an early pyramidal lesion above the level of C2 (but also in unilateral Parkinson's disease), the affected shoulder lags behind its fellow. Next, test deltoid, biceps, triceps, then the first dorsal interosseous and abductor pollicis brevis. In the lower limb, look at hip flexion and extension, knee flexion and extension and dorsiflexion and plantar flexion of the feet.

If the degree of muscle weakness fluctuates during the course of the examination, test for fatiguability.

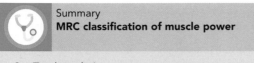

Summary
MRC classification of muscle power

0 Total paralysis
1 Flicker of contraction
2 Movement with gravity eliminated
3 Movement against gravity
4 Movement against resistance but incomplete
5 Normal power

Myotonia results in impaired relaxation of skeletal muscle after contraction. Ask the patient to clench the fists tightly then release them; if the patient has myotonia, there is a significant delay before the fingers can be fully extended. There is likely to be abnormal dimpling of muscle after percussion. Tap the thenar eminence with the patella hammer. In the presence of myotonia, the muscle dimples and stays dimpled for several seconds. The same sign can be elicited in the tongue.

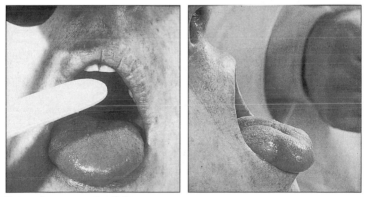

Percussion myotonia of the tongue.

DEEP TENDON REFLEXES
Testing the reflexes assesses the reflex arc and the supraspinal influences that operate on it. Each reflex is graded according to strength of response as shown in the summary box.

THE UPPER LIMB
The reflexes of the upper limb routinely tested are the biceps, triceps and supinator (the roots subserving each reflex are shown in brackets).

Summary
Grading reflexes

Grade	Definition
0	Absent
±	Present only with reinforcement
+	Just present
++	Brisk normal
+++	Exaggerated response

Biceps (C5/6)

The whole arm must be exposed when testing this reflex. Place the thumb or index finger of your left hand on the biceps tendon then strike it with the patella hammer using a pendular motion by extending then flexing your wrist. If there is no response, ask the patient to clench their teeth or grip the fingers of the other hand shortly before testing (Jendrassik manoeuvre). Now examine the reflex in the left arm.

Supinator (C5/6)

With the patient's arm in the semi-pronated position, strike the radial margin of the forearm approximately 5 cm above the wrist. You can if you wish interpose your finger. The response is a contraction of brachioradialis and biceps. In certain instances, despite a depression of the direct reflex, flexion of the fingers still occurs (inversion). This physical finding, usually due to cervical spondylosis, suggests the combination of a depression of the reflex arc at the C5/6 level, together with an exaggeration of reflexes at a lower level due to a co-existent pyramidal tract disorder.

Triceps (C6/7)

To test the right triceps jerk, bring the patient's right arm well across the body, with the elbow flexed at approximately 90° so that the triceps tendon is adequately exposed. Strike the tendon with the patella hammer. Having tested the reflex on the right, bring the left arm over and test the reflex on that side.

Finger (C8)

The finger jerk is usually present only when there is a pathological exaggeration of the reflexes. With the patient's arm pronated, exert slight pressure on the flexed fingers with the fingers of your left hand. Now strike the back of your own fingers with the hammer. A positive response leads to a brief flexion of the fingertips.

LOWER LIMB
Knee (L2/3/4)

To test the knee jerks insert your left arm underneath the patient's knees and flex them to approximately 60°. Tap first the right patella tendon and then the left. If one or both reflexes is particularly brisk, test for knee clonus by fitting your thumb and index finger along the upper border of the patella with the knee extended. Exert a sudden, downward stretch and maintain it. Any repetitive contraction of the quadriceps (i.e. clonus) even if only two or three beats, is strongly suggestive of a pyramidal tract disorder.

Ankle (S1)
The patient's leg is abducted and externally rotated at the hip, flexed at the knee and flexed at the ankle. If hip abduction is limited, rest the leg on its fellow to allow adequate access to the Achilles tendon. If the reflex is brisk, look for clonus. With the limb in the same position, forcibly dorsiflex the ankle and maintain that position. Three to four beats of symmetrical ankle clonus is acceptable in normal individuals but asymmetric or more sustained clonus is pathological.

OTHER REFLEXES
Abdominal responses
Lightly draw the end of an orange stick across the four segments of the abdomen around the umbilicus. Normally there is a reflex contraction in each segment.

Cremasteric reflex
The cremasteric reflex is elicited by stroking the upper inner aspect of the thigh. It is mediated through segments L1 and L2 and leads to retraction of the ipsilateral testicle.

Plantar response
The plantar response is elicited by applying firm pressure (use an orange stick) to the lateral aspect of the sole of the foot, moving from the heel to the base of the fifth toe, then, if necessary, across the base of the toes. While you do this observe the metatarsophalangeal joint of the big toe. In the normal adult, the toe plantar flexes. In the presence of a pyramidal tract lesion, the toe dorsiflexes. Summarise your findings with arrows: for flexor ↓, for extensor ↑ and for equivocal ↑↓.

Anal reflex
The anal reflex is assessed by pricking the skin at the anal margin. In normal people, there is a brisk contraction of the anal sphincter. The tone of the anal sphincter can be assessed by inserting a finger into the anus and asking the patient to bear down.

THE EXTRAPYRAMIDAL SYSTEM
Bradykinesia
Bradykinesia is particularly associated with Parkinson's disease. Initiation of movement is delayed, the actual movement slowed and its adjustment

insensitive. To look for bradykinesia in the upper limbs, ask the patient to tap repetitively the back of one hand with the other. Now ask the patient to 'polish' the back of one hand with the other. In bradykinesia, a movement of reduced amplitude is seen that eventually may cease completely. To assess bradykinesia in the lower limbs, ask the patient to tap your hand repetitively, first with one foot, then the other.

Involuntary movement
Begin by detailing the characteristics of the movement. Is it present at rest, with the limb completely supported or when the limb takes up a particular posture or only when the patient carries out a skilled activity?

Tremor
Tremor is a rhythmic movement that, at a particular joint, is usually confined to a single plane.

Myoclonus
Myoclonus is characterised by rapid, recurring muscle jerks.

Chorea
Patients with chorea appear to fidget. They show brief, random movements that do not have the shock-like quality of myoclonus. Both proximal and distal limb muscles can be affected.

Athetosis
Athetoid movements are slower still than chorea and become prominent during the performance of voluntary activity. The distal parts of the limbs are predominantly affected. In the hand, the posture oscillates between hyper-extension of the fingers and thumb, usually with pronation of the forearm and flexion of the digits associated with supination. In some patients, the movements are superimposed on more sustained postures.

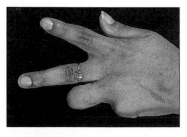

Athetoid hand posture.

Hemiballismus
Hemiballismus results in violent swinging movements of the contralateral arm and leg.

Dystonia

In dystonia, abnormal postures result from the contraction of antagonistic muscle groups.

Tics

Tics are repetitive movements that appear, at least briefly, to be under voluntary control. Typical examples are head nodding and jerking.

Dyskinesia

Brief, involuntary movements around the mouth and face are relatively common in elderly people (orofacial dyskinesia). Similar movements can be induced by long-term phenothiazine therapy and in patients on L-dopa.

Myokymia

Myokymia confined to the eyelid is a common experience in normal individuals and is felt as a fine twitching. In pathological myokymia, this fine movement extends to other parts of the facial musculature.

Asterixis

In certain metabolic disorders, particularly hepatic and renal failure, there is a defect of limb posture control. If the patient is asked to extend his or her arms and hold the fingers in the horizontal plane, a downward drift of the fingers and hands is interrupted by a sudden, upward, corrective jerk.

CLINICAL APPLICATION

UPPER MOTOR NEURON LESION

Summary
Features of upper motor neuron lesion

- Muscle weakness
- Increased deep tendon reflexes
- An extensor plantar response
- Depressed abdominal responses
- Spasticity

LOWER MOTOR NEURON LESION

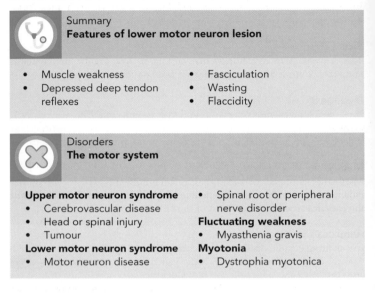

Summary
Features of lower motor neuron lesion

- Muscle weakness
- Depressed deep tendon reflexes
- Fasciculation
- Wasting
- Flaccidity

Disorders
The motor system

Upper motor neuron syndrome
- Cerebrovascular disease
- Head or spinal injury
- Tumour

Lower motor neuron syndrome
- Motor neuron disease

- Spinal root or peripheral nerve disorder

Fluctuating weakness
- Myasthenia gravis

Myotonia
- Dystrophia myotonica

Myasthenia gravis

In myasthenia gravis fatiguable weakness can affect any skeletal muscle. Diplopia and ptosis are particularly common. Muscle wasting is a late and inconsistent feature. The tendon reflexes are preserved.

EXTRAPYRAMIDAL DISORDERS

A combination of tremor, rigidity and bradykinesia occurs in Parkinson's disease. Postural problems are common; the neck and trunk become flexed. When walking, arm swing is reduced on one or both sides and turning is difficult, the patient taking more steps than usual. The Shy–Drager syndrome causes extrapyramidal features but also affects pyramidal, cerebellar and autonomic pathways. Many patients with rigidity and bradykinesia have had their symptoms induced by drugs affecting the release of dopamine or its receptor sites, for example, a phenothiazine. Another disorder affecting the extrapyramidal pathways disrupts first the supranuclear, then the nuclear, gaze pathways: the Steele–Richardson–Olsczewski syndrome (progressive supranuclear palsy).

MOVEMENT DISORDERS
Tremor

Essential (familial tremor) – Absent at rest. Can affect the head, neck and voice as well as the upper limbs and lower limbs.

Parkinsonian tremor – Classically a resting tremor at 4–5 Hz, with flexion–extension movements at the wrist and fingers, together with pronation–supination. Inhibited briefly by a skilled activity.

Myoclonus
Palatal myoclonus – Affects the palate, larynx and face. Frequency is 2–3 Hz. Associated with brainstem pathology, usually vascular.
Segmental myoclonus – Occurs with spinal cord disease.
Generalised myoclonus – Many causes.

Chorea
Sydenham's (rheumatic) chorea – Sometimes reappears in adult life, either spontaneously or during pregnancy.
Huntington's disease – Usually a prominent feature although not in juvenile-onset cases.
Other causes – Thyrotoxicosis, systemic lupus erythematosus, polycythaemia and the oral contraceptive pill.

Hemiballismus
Usually due to a vascular lesion in contralateral subthalamic nucleus.

Dystonia
Torsion dystonia – Familial, generalised dystonia predominating in either axial or limb muscles.
Drug-induced – e.g. dopa.
Focal dystonia – e.g. blepharospasm, spasmodic torticollis and writer's cramp.

Myokymia
Facial myokymia is associated with brainstem tumours and multiple sclerosis.

Summary
The motor system

- Inspect muscle bulk and assess any fasciculation
- Examine muscle tone
- Examine power using MRC classification
- Perform the deep tendon reflexes, along with the abdominal and plantar responses
- Assess any involuntary movement

THE CEREBELLAR SYSTEM

SYMPTOMS

Dysarthria

Patients with dysarthria have a defect of pronunciation, although speech content remains normal.

Limb clumsiness

A unilateral cerebellar disorder results in an ipsilateral limb ataxia. If the dominant limb is affected, the patient may well have noticed an alteration in writing. Sometimes the patient may refer to an ataxic limb as being weak rather than clumsy.

Gait ataxia

If the cerebellar problem is confined to one hemisphere, the patient often complains of deviating to that side when walking. With disruption of mid-line cerebellar structures, however, unsteadiness when walking is the main complaint rather than a tendency to deviate to a particular side.

EXAMINATION

SPEECH

In cerebellar dysarthria, speech volume and pitch are typically erratic, so that the rhythm of speech is lost, with pauses then accelerations. If the disorder is severe, speech is shot out in a staccato fashion.

EYE MOVEMENTS

In patients suspected of having cerebellar disease, you need to look for nystagmus and for abnormalities of either saccadic or pursuit movements.

Summary
Eye signs in cerebellar disease

Location	Sites
Flocculus	Abnormal smooth pursuit gaze-evoked nystagmus
Flocculus/nodulus	Down-beat nystagmus
Vermis/fastigial nucleus	Ocular dysmetria
Lateral zones	Ocular dysmetria gaze-evoked nystagmus

LIMB EXAMINATION

If there is a severe cerebellar disturbance, the outstretched hands may oscillate. More likely, however, is the presence of an intention tremor. To test this ask the patient to touch first his or her nose then your finger held approximately 0.5 m in front of him or her. In a cerebellar ataxia, a tremor emerges that becomes more apparent as the target is approached.

While testing for intention tremor, observe whether the patient's finger reaches the target accurately. It may reach beyond the target (hypermetria), fall short (hypometria) or even bounce against it in an uncontrolled fashion.

Now assess alternating movements in the upper limbs. Ask the patient to raise his or her arms rapidly from the sides but to stop them abruptly in the horizontal plane. In cerebellar disease, the affected arm oscillates about its intended resting place because of a failure of the damping mechanism.

To assess lower limb co-ordination, ask the patient to slide the heel of one foot in a straight line down the shin of the other leg: the heel–knee–shin test. In the presence of cerebellar ataxia the heel wavers around the intended pathway.

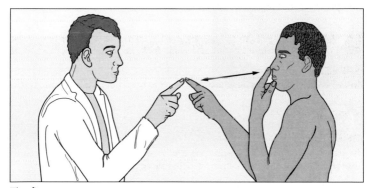

The finger–nose test.

GAIT

When walking, the patient will use a wide-based gait and is likely to show caution when turning. If the patient has a lesion of one cerebellar hemisphere, then deviation to that side occurs on walking.

LESIONS OF THE CEREBELLAR HEMISPHERE
The lesions most commonly affecting the cerebellar hemisphere are infarcts, haemorrhage and tumour.

MIDLINE CEREBELLAR LESIONS
The predominant complaint in patients with lesions of the vermis or paravermis is a gait ataxia. The familial cerebellar atrophies tend to produce a more diffuse atrophy readily detectable by CT scanning.

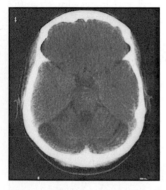

CT scan showing diffuse cerebellar atrophy.

Disorders
Cerebellum

Hemisphere lesions
- Stroke
- Primary and secondary tumours
- Multiple sclerosis

- Degenerative disorders

Vermis lesions
- Alcohol-related
- Hypothyroidism

Summary
Cerebellar system examination

- Assess articulation
- Examine pursuit and saccadic eye movements and analyse any nystagmus
- Examine the finger–nose and heel–knee–shin tests
- Assess gait

THE SENSORY SYSTEM

Summary
Sensory disturbances

	Light touch	**Pain**
Reduced	Hypaesthesia	Hypalgesia
Lost	Anaesthesia	Analgesia
Exaggerated	Hyperaesthesia	Hyperpathia
Exaggerated (at normal threshold)	–	Hyperalgesia

SYMPTOMS

Sensory symptoms include pain, paraesthesiae (tingling) and numbness.

PAIN

Only rarely does the particular quality of a pain serve to identify its likely source. In peripheral nerve injury, signs of nerve damage may be accompanied by a distressing, persistent burning sensation known as causalgia. A particular type of pain can emerge after damage to the spinothalamic tract or the thalamus itself (thalamic pain). It is persistent, with a very unpleasant burning or scalding quality and is exacerbated by painful or tactile contact.

PARAESTHESIAE AND NUMBNESS

Patients often struggle when describing the nature of sensory disturbances.

Questions to ask
Sensory disturbances

- When the patient describes numbness, does he or she mean actual loss of cutaneous sensation?
- Does the distribution of any numbness or tingling follow the distribution of a peripheral nerve or nerve root?
- Does the patient describe loss or altered sensation ascending onto the abdomen or thorax?

EXAMINATION

Sensory examination is difficult. There are few objective criteria, assessment being largely dependent on the patient's subjective responses that may well falter as the patient fatigues. If the patient has an area of reduced cutaneous sensation, start testing within that area, moving out gradually to determine the zone of transition to normal sensation.

LIGHT TOUCH

Use a wisp of cotton wool to test light touch sensation. Do not drag the cotton wool along the surface of the skin but apply it at a single point. Ask the patient to close his or her eyes and to respond when contact is made.

In parietal lesions, the half-body supplied by the damaged cortex may fail to register a stimulus when there is competition from the intact opposite side, even though a stimulus, applied in isolation, is appreciated (sensory suppression or extinction).

TWO-POINT DISCRIMINATION

Two-point discrimination is tested with a pair of compasses specifically designed for this purpose, with gradations in centimetres indicating the separation of the tips. As an approximate guide, a young adult will detect a separation of approximately 3 mm on the finger tips, 1 cm on the palm of the hand and 3 cm on the sole of the foot.

PROPRIOCEPTION

While assessing joint position sense ensure that the patient's eyes remain closed. During testing avoid pressing on the digit in such a way that the patient appreciates the direction of movement. To test the terminal interphalangeal joint of the index finger grip, the sides of the phalanx with the thumb and forefinger of your right hand using your left to stabilise the proximal joints of the finger. If the responses are inaccurate, move proximally until the movements are accurately perceived.

You can test active proprioception by asking the patient with the eyes closed to locate a digit of one hand with the index finger of the other limb. Finally, ask the patient to hold the hands outstretched while the eyes are closed. With severe loss of distal proprioception, the fingers move in an irregular, purposeless fashion, as if exploring their environment (pseudo-athetosis).

To test the quality of the proprioceptive information coming from the lower limbs, ask the patient to stand with their feet together and their eyes closed. Where there is loss of proprioception, the patient immediately loses stability (positive Romberg's test).

VIBRATION SENSE

Vibration sense is tested using a 128 Hz tuning fork. To test in the finger, apply the gently vibrating base of the fork to the pulp of the finger or the knuckle of the distal interphalangeal joint. For the foot, start with the pad of the big toe or the dorsum of the interphalangeal joint. If vibration sense is absent there, test more proximally.

PAIN
Pain is best tested using a sharp pin or needle. Purpose made 'sharps' are now available which should be discarded using standard safety procedures after use.

Deep pain sense can be tested by applying pressure to deeper structures, for example, by pinching the tendo Achilles.

TEMPERATURE
To test temperature sense it generally suffices to use two metal tubes, one containing water mixed with ice chips, the other containing hot water. Test the tubes on yourself before testing the patient.

WEIGHT, SHAPE, SIZE AND TEXTURE
Certain sensory modalities are worth testing if a disturbance of cortical function is suspected. To test weight appreciation put an object in the patient's palm, allowing the hand to move up and down so that the patient appreciates both the pressure exerted by the weight and the resistance experienced when the hand is moved against gravity.

Shape recognition is also heavily dependent on cortical function. Ask the patient to assess the shape of a coin and also (although this involves other sensory modalities) whether it possesses a milled edge. You can use materials of different form (velvet, wool, linen and so on) to test the patient's appreciation of texture.

CLINICAL APPLICATION

NERVE AND ROOT DISORDERS
Within an affected nerve or root distribution all sensory modalities will be equally affected, with a boundary zone of partial loss in which appreciation of light touch is more disturbed than that of pain and temperature. If pain fibres to the skin and joints are affected, consequences include painless skin ulceration, sometimes leading to amputation or a severe derangement of joint function.

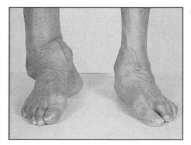

Charcot joint. Right ankle.

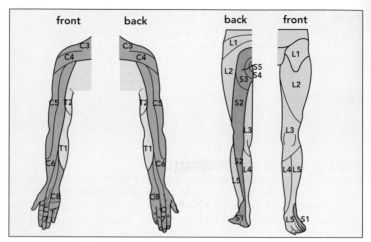

Dermatomes of the upper and lower limbs.

SPINAL CORD DISORDERS

Transverse cord lesion – Sensory level around the site of the lesion often with a small zone in which cutaneous stimulation can evoke a painful reaction.

Unilateral cord lesion (Brown–Séquard) – Produces contralateral loss of pain and temperature to a level slightly below the lesion, with ipsilateral weakness, depression of vibration and joint position sense.

Central cord lesion – Disrupts crossing spinothalamic fibres leading to bilateral, selective loss of pain and temperature over the affected segments.

Dorsal column lesion – Interferes with vibration sense, proprioception and two-point discrimination. Some patients with cervical dorsal column lesions describe a shock-like sensation radiating down the spine when the neck is flexed (Lhermitte's sign).

External compression – Tends to spare the deeper fibres in the spinothalamic tract coming from the segments immediately below the level of compression. Brainstem and thalamic disorders – In the medulla, lateral lesions predominantly affect contralateral pain and temperature sensation, whereas medial lesions disrupt sensation served by the dorsal columns. Thalamic lesions affect all aspects of sensation on the opposite side of the body.

CORTICAL LESIONS

It allows definition of object size, shape, weight and texture. Loss of this facility is called astereognosis. The cortex allows both accurate definition of the site of contact and discrimination of single or multiple stimulation. It is closely concerned with the appreciation of joint position. Sensory suppression is a particular feature of cortical lesions. In nondominant parietal lobe lesions, neglect of the contralateral limbs can be so profound that the patient denies their existence and tries to remove them as if belonging to another person.

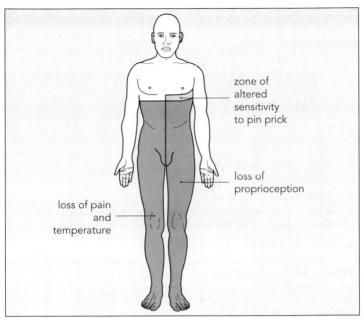

Distribution of sensory and deficit in Brown–Séquard lesion.

NONORGANIC SENSORY LOSS

The most common pattern of nonorganic sensory loss is one in which cutaneous sensation to all modalities is affected, with little or no change in proprioception. Typically, a single limb is involved but sometimes the problem occupies one side or the lower half of the body.

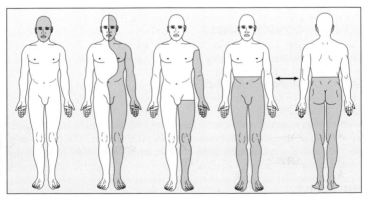

Patterns of nonorganic sensory loss.

THE UNCONSCIOUS PATIENT

SYMPTOMS

Coma is the consequence either of extensive bilateral hemisphere disease, a unilateral hemisphere mass lesion or a more discrete pathology confined to certain parts of the brainstem.

Mass lesions in one cerebral hemisphere affect the conscious level by causing downward herniation of brain tissue through the tentorial notch, with secondary compression of the brainstem. Two types of herniation are described, a central form, usually associated with slowly expanding, medially placed masses and an uncal form, in which masses in the middle cranial fossa, particularly of the temporal lobe, cause displacement of the medial aspect of the uncus over the free edge of the tentorium.

EXAMINATION

SKELETAL SYSTEM

Palpate the long bones for evidence of fracture. Note the presence of any localised scalp swelling indicating focal trauma and inspect the external auditory meati for signs of bleeding, suggesting the possibility of a basal skull fracture.

CARDIOVASCULAR SYSTEM

Perform a routine cardiovascular assessment.

RESPIRATORY SYSTEM

Assess respiratory rhythm and rate.

GASTROINTESTINAL SYSTEM

Palpate the abdomen. Look for other markers of liver disease, such as spider naevi.

LEVEL OF CONSCIOUSNESS

Having performed other aspects of the examination, you can then proceed to grade the conscious level using the Glasgow Coma Scale.

SIGNS OF MENINGEAL IRRITATION

Flex the neck to see whether there is any abnormal resistance to the movement or a reaction on the part of the patient. Neck stiffness suggests meningeal irritation. Kernig's test is performed by flexing the leg at the hip with the knee flexed, then extending the leg at the knee. The patient may react as the leg is extended or there may be an obvious reflex spasm in the hamstring muscles.

THE PUPILS

Examine the pupils for symmetry and size then test the direct light response

	Patient's response	Score	08.00	10.00	12.00
Eye opening	spontaneous	4			
	to speech	3			
	to pain	2			
	none	1			
Best verbal responses	orientated	5			
	confused	4			
	inappropriate	3			
	incomprehensible	2			
	none	1			
Best motor responses	obeying	6			
	localising	5			
	withdrawing	4			
	flexing	3			
	extending	2			
	none	1			

Glasgow coma scale.

using a bright pencil torch. Disruption of the third nerve beyond the nucleus produces a characteristic eye position associated with a fixed dilated pupil.

In metabolic coma, the pupils remain reactive and symmetric although often relatively small. Certain drugs can influence pupil size or reactivity. Atropine will cause pupillary dilatation, as will over-dosage of amphetamines or tricyclic anti-depressants. Morphine derivatives, in excessive dosage, result in pinpoint pupils that retain their reactivity.

OCULAR MOVEMENTS

First note any spontaneous eye movements. Now assess eye movements. Having gently elevated the upper lids, firmly rotate the head laterally, then vertically (doll's head manoeuvre). If reflex eye movements are intact, the eyes move so as to leave them directed forwards. A more potent stimulus for reflex eye movement is achieved by caloric stimulation.

Sustained horizontal ocular deviation indicates a frontal or brainstem lesion. In the former, the eyes deviate away from the side of the accompanying hemiplegia. In a brainstem lesion below the decussation of the supranuclear pathway for horizontal gaze, the eyes deviate to the opposite side and hence to the side of an accompanying hemiparesis.

MOTOR RESPONSES

Motor function in the limbs can be assessed partly by observing the patient's posture and partly by assessing the response to pressure over the sternum or, for assessing the limb response, squeezing the nail bed of a digit or the tendo Achilles. The two principal inappropriate responses are decorticate and decerebrate posturing. In the former, the upper limbs flex and adduct, the lower limbs extend and plantar flex. In decerebrate rigidity, the upper limbs are extended, adducted and hyperpronated, with the lower limbs fully extended.

RESPIRATORY STATUS

A number of abnormal respiratory patterns in the unconscious patient may allow localisation of the lesion responsible for the coma.

CLINICAL APPLICATION

METABOLIC COMA

The pupils remain reactive until the late stages of metabolic coma. The eyes remain central but reflex movement, even that elicited by caloric stimulation, may eventually be lost. Both generalised and focal motor seizures occur. Decorticate or decerebrate posturing are seen. In drug–induced coma, although the doll's head and cold caloric responses are eventually lost, the pupils usually remain reactive until the very late stages.

STRUCTURAL CAUSES OF COMA

With central herniation, as the conscious state alters, the first eye movement abnormality observed is impairment of reflex upward gaze. The pupils remain reactive. As a hemisphere lesion is present, there is likely to be a contralateral hemiplegia. Further signs appear as the transtentorial herniation proceeds. Horizontal eye movements become increasingly difficult to elicit, even using caloric stimulation. The pupils become fixed to light but remain midposition in size. Decorticate posturing of the unaffected side becomes decerebrate.

Uncal herniation produces a different picture, at least initially. The pupil of the eye ipsilateral to the lesion becomes dilated and this is followed by the development of an ophthalmoplegia. Initially, the contralateral pupil remains reactive and the eye moves fully with reflex stimulation but subsequently reflex movements are lost. The limbs ipsilateral to the lesion can develop a hemiplegic

Disorders
Causes of coma

Metabolic coma
- Hypoglycaemia
- Hyperglycaemia
- Uraemia
- Hepatic encephalopathy
- Hypercapnoea
- Drug-induced coma

Structural coma
- Hemisphere mass lesions: tumour, extra-dural haematoma, sub-dural haematoma, brainstem stroke

posture relatively early, due to compression of the contralateral cerebral peduncle against the tentorial edge. Later bilateral decerebrate posturing appears.

The final stages of the two types of herniation are similar.

Supratentorial masses producing coma are usually vascular rather than neoplastic.

BRAIN DEATH

The end point of many structural and metabolic insults to the brain is a state in which a deeply comatose patient maintains circulatory function providing that respiration is supported by artificial means. There is good evidence to suggest that if brainstem function can be shown to have ceased in such patients, there is no prospect for recovery. Criteria of brainstem death have been devised to appraise this state, in order to identify patients in whom further attempts at life-support are of no value.

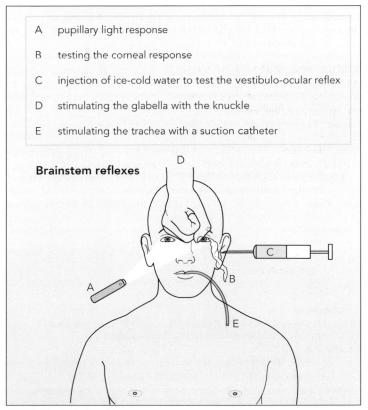

A   pupillary light response

B   testing the corneal response

C   injection of ice-cold water to test the vestibulo-ocular reflex

D   stimulating the glabella with the knuckle

E   stimulating the trachea with a suction catheter

Brainstem reflexes

Testing brainstem reflexes.

Summary
Examination of the unconscious patient

- Assess conscious level
- Examine for signs of meningeal irritation
- Pupils
- Ocular movements
- Motor responses and reflexes
- Respiration

Examination of elderly people
The nervous system

Primitive reflexes
- Glabellar tap – Found with increasing frequency with age
- Palmo-mental reflex – Bilateral responses found with increasing frequency with age
- Snout and suckling reflexes – Seldom, particularly the latter, found in normal, elderly individuals
- Grasp reflex – The presence of grasp reflexes correlates with evidence of cognitive impairment

Cranial nerve function
- Smell – Sensitivity declines after the age of 65 years
- Eyes
  - Mild ptosis common in elderly people
  - Upgaze declines with age
  - The light and accommodation responses decline with age and the pupils become more miosed
- Taste – Sensitivity declines with age, with a higher threshold
- Hearing – Declines with age

Motor system
- Reflexes
  - Contrary to established teaching, the ankle jerks are preserved in old age
  - The abdominal responses diminish and their latency increases with age
- Movements
  - Lingual–facial–buccal dyskinesias are found in elderly people without a history of neuroleptic drug exposure

Sensation
- Vibration – Threshold for appreciation increases with age
- Two-point discrimination – Threshold increases with age

Gait
- Becomes increasingly cautious with increasing age

12. Infants and Children

The general principles of history taking and examination still apply, but the manner and order in which they are approached differ and the emphasis is different in children. There are five age bands to consider:

- Newborn and very young baby (0–8 weeks)
- Older baby and toddler (2–24 months)
- Preschool child (2–5 years)
- School child (5–10+ years)
- Adolescent (10 to approximately 16 years).

TAKING A HISTORY

Listen to the parents and, generally, if they describe a problem then there is a diagnosis to be made. In the younger child you will be more reliant on the parents' account.

The older the child, the more you can communicate with them. Try and allow the child (including the siblings) to feel relaxed and comfortable during the consultation; this is more likely if there are a variety of toys and games lying about the room. Children up to and including school age may well prefer to be on a parent's lap.

The family history is important and can be clearly presented by using a three-generation family tree. The family tree can be further annotated helping to fill in details of the child's social history.

Child abuse is a common problem. Children can be harmed by adults in a number of different ways: emotionally, physically, sexually, by neglect or, rarely, by induced illnesses and poisoning. The nature of any injury or illness in any child, from any background, must be explained satisfactorily in the history and be a plausible cause of the findings seen on examination. If you have any such concerns about a child or family you must share them with colleagues and social services.

THE EXAMINATION

Inspection and observation are the most important. The younger the child, the more important it is to observe the child's wellbeing and any physical signs from a distance. Do not wake up sleeping children to examine them until you have observed them carefully first.

The younger the child, the more imaginative one may have to be to ensure a satisfactory consultation but remember it is easy to make older children and adolescents feel patronised.

Try not to allow your eye level to be much higher than that of your patient. Always remember what it's like from the child's perspective.

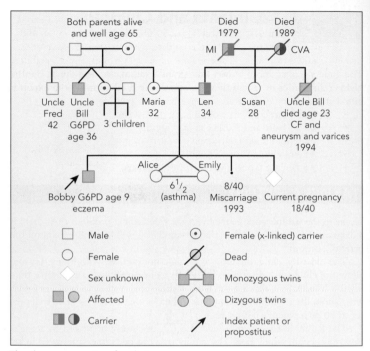

The three-generation family tree.

It may take time to win the confidence of young children. The pyrexial, irritable child may not allow you any physical contact without crying despite a friendly approach. With palpation and auscultation the order in which you perform them depends on where the problem is, what the problem is likely to be and how ill and how co-operative the patient is. When possible, start peripherally making it clear to the child that you are a friendly doctor. Percussion is rarely a rewarding process in the very young. Young patients should think the examination is fun. Avoid unpleasant procedures if at all possible (e.g. rectal examinations).

GROWTH AND DEVELOPMENT

A continuum of growth from baby to adult has been described by three main phases:
- The infant phase: a continuation of the foetal growth rate that slows down into the second year. The critical factors in this phase are nutrition and hormones controlling metabolism.
- The childhood phase: from the second to beyond the 10th year. The critical factors in this phase are the pituitary hormones (e.g. growth hormone).

- The adolescent phase: extends from puberty until the achievement of final adult stature. The critical factors in this phase are the sex steroids.

Any examination of a child is incomplete without an assessment of their growth and development. Assess weight in all ages, supine length and head circumference in infants (under the age of 2 years), and standing height in older children. Growth charts are used to help to determine the expected range at any given age.

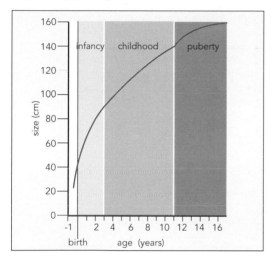

Three phases of growth in childhood (after Karlberg).

DEVELOPMENT

The evaluation of development is complicated. There is a large variation in the normal patterns of development.

For convenience, development is usually considered under eight main headings, which can be easily remembered as four sets of pairs:

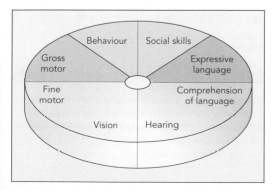

All these areas are dependent on each other. Some doctors group hearing & speech and vision & fine motor together, reflecting this interdependence.

THE NEWBORN AND VERY YOUNG BABY

Summary
Gestation and weight of gestation

- Preterm – born before 37 completed weeks' gestation from last menstrual period (LMP)
- Term – born between 37 and 42 completed weeks' gestation from LMP
- Post-term – born after 42 completed weeks' gestation from LMP
- Small for gestational age or 'small for dates' – birth weight below 10th centile for gestational age
- Large for gestational age or 'large for dates' – birth weight greater than 90th centile for gestational age

Newborns and young babies are examined routinely at birth, at 6 weeks of age and when receiving immunisations.

The very young (like the very old) often have nonspecific symptoms and signs even when they are seriously ill. To help, a scoring system for symptoms and signs was developed: 'Baby Check'.

Newborns and young babies can become very sick quickly. Infection should be included in the differential diagnosis of any sick baby.

Baby Check total scores

0-7 Baby is only a little unwell, medical attention is not necessary.

8-12 Baby is unwell but not seriously, seek advise from doctor, health visitor or midwife.

13-19 Baby is ill, contact your doctor and arrange to be seen.

>20 Baby is seriously ill and needs to see a doctor immediately.

If the baby appears to be worse after a low score, then re-examine the baby and rescore.

Baby check is a system to help parents, health professionals and carers to assess the seriousness of a baby's illness. It uses 19 signs and symptoms and scores when added together give a total. The total score correlates with the seriousness of the baby's illness. The scoring system has been validated for use by parents, doctors and nurses in babies under 6 months old. Adapted from 'Baby Check' booklet.

1. Unusual cry	e.g. high pitched, weak, moaning or painful	Score 2
2. Fluids taken in previous 24 hours	Less than normal Half normal Very little	Score 2 Score 4 Score 9
3. Vomiting	Vomiting at least half of a feed in the three previous feeds	Score 4
4. Vomiting bile	Any green bile in vomit	Score 13
5. Wet nappies (urine output)	Less urine than normal	Score 3
6. Blood in nappy	Large amount of blood in nappy	Score 11
7. Drowsiness	Occasionally drowsy Drowsy most of the time	Score 3 Score 5
8. Floppiness	Baby seems more floppy than normal	Score 4
9. Watching	Baby less watchful than normal	Score 2
10. Awareness	Baby responding less than normally to their surroundings	Score 2
11. Breathing difficulties	Minimal recession visible Obvious recession visible	Score 4 Score 15
12. Looking pale	Baby more pale than normal, or been pale in last 24 h	Score 3
13. Wheezing	Baby has wheezy breathing sounds	Score 2
14. Blue nails	Apparent blue nails	Score 3
15. Circulation	Baby's toes are white, or stay white for three s after squeezing	Score 3
16. Rash	Rash over body, or raw, weeping area >5 x 5cm	Score 4
17. Hernia	Obvious bulge in scrotum or groin	Score 13
18. Temperature (rectal)	Temperature is >38.3°C by rectal thermometer	Score 4
19. Crying during checks	If baby has cried during checks (more than a grizzle)	Score 4

GROWTH

Newborns tend to lose from 5 to 10% of their birth weight in the first week but then steadily gain an average of 25–30 g per day over the next 6 months. Head circumference is a valuable measurement.

DEVELOPMENT
Behaviour observed in neonates is the result of responses initiated by the brainstem and spinal cord, for example, startling to sound and the primitive reflexes.

HISTORY
Feeding history is important, it is the most strenuous activity the newborn has to do. Compromise in cardiorespiratory function is revealed in difficulty in taking or completing feeds. Details about maternal health, the pregnancy and delivery, as well as the baby's condition and birth weight, should be noted.

EXAMINATION
Circulation and cardiovascular system
• Normal heart rate ranges are 110–160 beats/min (>180 tachycardia).
• Normal systolic blood pressure ranges are 65–110 mmHg (depends on age). Auscultation of the heart sounds and listening for murmurs may be the priority before the baby cries. Central cyanosis is observed on the mucous membranes.

Difficulty in palpating or absent femoral pulses should be followed up with four-limb blood pressure measurements to exclude coarctation of the aorta. Large volume pulses are found with a patent ductus arteriosus. The apex beat should be palpated and the presence of thrills noted.

Systolic murmurs are common in the newborn (greater than 20% babies on day 1) and not all are due to congenital heart lesions. Pansystolic, continuous murmurs and ejection systolic murmurs that radiate to the back or neck are suspicious. Many babies with structural congenital heart disease may not have a murmur, although they may have symptoms and other signs of cardiovascular disease.

Abdomen
Observing a feed and inspection of stools can be important parts of the evaluation. Vomiting is common, but bile-stained vomiting warrants urgent assessment.

Questions to ask
Jaundice in young babies

• Was the baby jaundiced in the first 24 h of life?
• Was the baby still jaundiced during the third week of life?
• Is the baby well?
• What are the colour of the stools and the urine?

Jaundice from the third to 10th day is very common and usually physiological. Jaundice in the first 24 h of life is pathological until proven otherwise.

After 2-weeks' old jaundice is usually related to breastfeeding but if associated with pale stools, failure to thrive or a green tint to the jaundice, then a pathological cause is more likely.

The palate is inspected for clefts and palpated for submucous clefts. The position and patency of the anus needs to be checked. The external genitalia should be inspected. In boys, both testes should be in the scrotum. Small hydrocoeles are common and need no action. If hernias are suspected then refer to a paediatric surgeon. The penis should have a normally sited urethral orifice with a foreskin adherent to the glans (this adherence is physiological and should not be interfered with). In girls there should be an introitus and a normally sized clitoris. Any ambiguity in the genitalia requires urgent assessment by a paediatric endocrinologist before sex is assigned.

The umbilical stump has usually separated by the 10th day.

A liver edge is usually palpable (approximately 1 cm below the costal margin) and the lower pole of the right kidney and a spleen tip are sometimes palpable.

Examine the hips using the Ortolani and Barlow manoeuvres to detect abnormalities in the hip joint.

Breathing and respiration

- Normal respiratory rate ranges are 30–50 breaths/min (>60 tachypnoea). The presence of respiratory distress is an important observation. Auscultatory signs are less significant than the observations.

All babies are obligate nose-breathers (during feeding) and nasal obstruction may be related to feeding difficulties. The presence of audible inspiratory stridor as a finding warrants further evaluation.

> Summary
> **Respiratory distress (the combination of some or all of the following)**
>
> - Tachypnoea (normal upper limit varies with age)
> - Recession (includes subcostal, intercostal or tracheal tug)
> - Grunting (an end expiratory groaning noise, breathing out against partially adducted vocal cords and providing self positive end expiratory pressure)
> - Flaring of nostrils (the alae nasi are accessory muscles of respiration)
> - Cyanosis (may be subclinical – check O_2 saturation with pulse oximeter)

Neurology and development

The fontanelle's tone is altered by crying. Wide fontanelles, especially the posterior, may be related to delayed skeletal maturation (many causes) or the possibility of raised intracranial pressure. A cranial ultrasound scan will quick-ly rule out enlarged ventricles.

Moulding or caput is common in the first 24 h as is a chignon after a ven-touse delivery. Swelling over either parietal bones is usually caused by cephalohaematomas (subperiosteal bleeds). The head circumference should be measured.

The best way to assess a newborn's nervous system is to observe the baby. Eliciting all the primitive reflexes is less helpful than observation. The asymmetric tonic neck reflex is a strong influence on posture and movement. The Moro (startle) reflex is an unpleasant stimulus to the baby and should not be done without a good reason. The baby should be able to fix on and fol-low an object through 90°. Use an ophthalmoscope to look for the presence of a red reflex in each eye. Young babies startle to loud noises.

THE ROUTINE NEONATAL EXAMINATION

Developed countries have a policy of examining all neonates in the first few days of life.

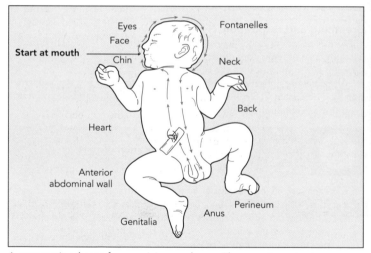

A systematic scheme for examining newborns. The more important congenital anomalies tend to occur on or near the midline, so using a constant point of origin (e.g. the mouth) start examining the neonate along the midline, circumnavigating the entire baby and arriving back at your point of origin. At some points you may stray from the midline (e.g. to look at the eyes, or auscultate the heart). At the end do not forget the hands, feet and hips need checking.

Examine neonates in front of the parents. This examination, more than any other at a later date, is likely to reveal congenital abnormalities. Single minor congenital abnormalities occur with a frequency of up to 14% of live births. The greater the number of congenital abnormalities, the greater the possibility that there may be more serious congenital abnormalities present. Severe and lethal congenital abnormalities are seen in about 1.5% of live births.

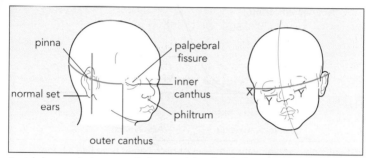

Facial dysmorphology vocabulary explained. A baby's face when viewed from the front, with a line through the eyes is about halfway from vertex to chin (X). Palpebral fissures (the slits through which your eyes look) should be of equal length (Y) measured from inner to outer canthus. There is usually a very mild slant to the palpebral fissures, if this slant is exaggerated then it is described as upward slanting. The slant may be in the opposite direction and is described as downward slanting. The distance between the eyes is approximately that of the palpebral fissures (Y). Hypotelorism is when (Y) is too short and hypertelorism is when (Y) is too long. A line from the outer canthus towards the occiput should cross the attachment of the upper helix of the pinna (ear lobe) to the side of the head. Where this does not occur then the ear is described as low set and may appear simple (poorly formed helix) and rotated as well.

OLDER BABIES AND TODDLERS

The term 'infant' has been used previously to describe children under 2 years of age.

There are very rapid changes in growth and especially in development. The effects of passively acquired maternal immunity start to decline (this means that babies are more prone to intercurrent viral illnesses). On average, the healthy baby and toddler will have to deal with eight intercurrent self-limiting viral illnesses per year.

In most countries, a comprehensive immunisation programme aims to prevent up to eight important diseases.

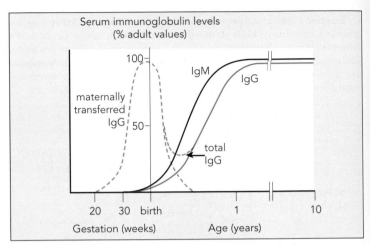

Immunoglobulin levels vary with age. At birth babies have had a trans-placental transfusion of maternal IgG that wears off by the end of the first 6 months. This provides passive immunity to the newborn; afterwards the child must develop their own active immunity after infection or immunisation.

GROWTH

Babies in this phase are still growing rapidly but there is a distinct decelera-tion in their growth velocity. The 'average baby' will have doubled their birth weight by approximately 5 months and trebled it by just after a year.

The dramatic changes in head growth are a result of myelination of cor-tical tracts and pathways leading to brain growth, which makes the develop-mental advances in this period possible.

DEVELOPMENT

The key question in this age group is whether the parents are concerned about their child's developmental progress.

HISTORY

The history should cover current feeding, weaning, developmental abilities and immunisations received.

EXAMINATION

Keep the child on the parent's lap and play with him or her. Show the child that whatever you are going to do is more of a game rather than anything more threatening. Examine the most relevant system indicated by the histo-ry first because this may be your only chance.

Circulation and cardiovascular system

• Normal heart rate ranges are 110–160 beats/min (>180 tachycardia).

• Normal systolic blood pressure ranges are 75–115 mmHg (depends on age). Capillary refill time should be the same as for adults (less than 2 to 3 s). Environmental cold stress can prolong the capillary refill time in otherwise well babies. Tachycardia in the absence of crying usually means some sort of stress.

Blood pressure should be measured in any sick infant or when cardiovascular, renal, endocrine or neurological diagnoses are being considered. The cuff size is critical as blood pressure measurements may be spuriously high if too small a cuff is used or the infant is crying. Normal ranges are published according to size and age.

> **Summary**
> **Children's blood pressure measurements can be obtained using:**
>
> • oscillometry (dynamapp)
> • sphygmomanometry (using a stethoscope or Doppler probe or by palpation)
> • direct (invasive) measurement (in intensive care)
> **Remember the two-thirds rule:**
> • cuff (bladder) width must be at least two-thirds of the distance from shoulder to elbow
> • cuff length must be at least two-thirds of the limb circumference

One-third of children will have a murmur heard at some point of their lives. Less than 1% of children will have a structural heart lesion. Innocent murmurs have particular characteristics: ejection systolic flow murmurs are either 'short and buzzing' (caused by turbulent aortic flow) or 'soft and blowing' (caused by turbulent pulmonary flow); venous hums are low pitched and more noticeable after exertion or inspiration and they are abolished by lying supine.

True pathological murmurs are usually louder, harsher and longer and can radiate. Other features are the presence of a diastolic component: symptoms and signs of cardiovascular disease.

Abdomen

After careful inspection, palpate with warm hands. Patience is needed and much more than one attempt at palpation may be required, perhaps when the child is sleeping on a parent's lap.

The hip joint may be a cause for concern because of an acquired limp. With the child on the parent's lap, gently explore the passive range of movements. Internal and external rotation of the hip (with the hip and knee both in 90° of flexion) is a sensitive way to pick up hip joint pathology.

Breathing and respiration

• Normal respiratory rate ranges are 20–40 breaths/min (>50 tachypnoea) Observing the child's respiratory pattern is the most useful part of the examination. Auscultation may add some more information, but is frequently 'drowned' by loud transmitted upper respiratory tract breath sounds.

Coryza (profuse nasal and pink inflamed mucous membranes in the throat and ears) is most likely to be caused by a viral upper respiratory tract infection.

Lymphadenopathy (localised or generalised) is common in association with frequent upper respiratory tract infections and viral illnesses. Acutely tender lymphadenopathy is associated with bacterial infections. Asymmetrical large (sometimes tender) lymphadenopathy with constitutional symptoms warrants further evaluation.

❌ Disorders
Rashes

Rashes in childhood are very common and all you need is a simple and logical approach to make a diagnosis most of the time.

- The most clinically important rashes to recognise promptly are ones that are purpuric (nonblanching), for examples refer to images below and on next page.
- If the rash is erythematous (blanching) and is associated with an intercurrent illness, then it is most probably related to an infection; often viral and self-limiting.
- Any chronically itchy rash is likely to be eczema and should be treated with emollients.

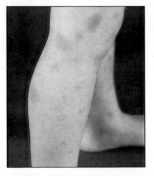

Idiopathic thrombocytopaenic purpura in childhood differs from the adult condition by being more benign and is self-limiting. Acute leukaemia is an important differential diagnosis to be excluded.

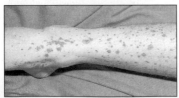

Henoch–Schönlein purpura is an 'allergic' vasculitis that has a characteristic distribution. It is associated with many systemic symptoms and (uncommonly) can result in permanent renal impairment.

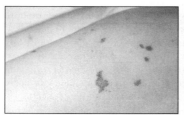

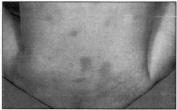

The lives of patients with meningococcal disease depend on their doctor recognising this purpuric rash as early as possible. It may start off as erythematous and non-blanching. It is the speed of the rash's progression that is a useful sign. Treat immediately with an appropriate parenteral antibiotic.

Fingertip bruising seen in non-accidental injury. All children have falls and minor injuries that result in bruises in areas of likely accidental impact (e.g. shins and elbows). Any bruise in a usually protected site is a worry. Ask how it happened? Is the injury consistent with the history? If you are worried, discuss immediately with qualified staff.

Neurology and development

Neurological assessment of infants relies on history (for developmental skills) and inspection and observation for confirmation of the reported abilities and the presence of any focal signs. When dealing with fits or 'funny turns', a first hand account is best of all. **Observation is most important.** Save cranial nerve examination until last and check behaviour, movement, gait and co-ordination by observation while the child plays.

Assess truncal tone in the youngest of babies upwards. Limbs are inspected and palpated in play to ascertain tone, muscle bulk, power and sensation. Deep tendon reflexes are elicited patiently; reinforcement is employed in play (squeeze the toy) if necessary. Co-ordination is hard to test, observation is the most one can do.

The cranial nerves

The first nerve Smell can be assessed by asking the toddler to find a mint hidden in a handkerchief.

The second nerve Visual acuity can be checked by a variety of techniques. Visual fields and employing fundoscopy are seldom possible in this age group without specialist equipment in younger infants. However, in the older (preschool age) child this is more straightforward and acuity can be checked beyond the age of two with shape or letter matching.

The third, fourth and sixth nerves Eye movements can be observed when the child follows a toy or light in the vertical and horizontal plane.

The fifth and seventh nerves The fifth nerve can be tested when the jaws are clenched on a bottle or biscuit; the sixth by encouraging the child to smile or shut the eyes.

The eighth nerve Hearing is routinely screened in children from 7–8 months.
The ninth, 10th, 11th and 12th nerves These nerves are more difficult to assess in this age group. Inspect the throat (at the end of your examination), the following can be seen: movement of the uvula as you inspect the throat (ninth nerve intact); no hoarseness in the cry (10th nerve intact); shrugging of the shoulders and turning of the head using the sternomastoid (11th nerve intact); waggling of the tongue as the spatula is used (12th nerve intact).

THE PRESCHOOL CHILD

GROWTH
It should be possible to estimate midparental height centile and compare it with the child's height centile.

Summary
Midparental height

- This calculation enables a prediction of the child's adult target height range
- The mean difference in final adult height is 13 cm between men and women
- For boys add 13 cm to mother's height
- For girls subtract 13 cm from father's height
- The midpoint between the parent's corrected heights is the midparental height
- For this there is a normal centile range

DEVELOPMENT
This is characterised by advances in communication and the use and understanding of language. Social and behavioural landmarks include the general behaviour as well as specific abilities, e.g. potty training.

HISTORY
The history should include details about developmental skills acquired and whether the parents or health visitor have any concerns. Specific points include diet (peak age), exercise tolerance and coughing.

EXAMINATION
Generally this is best done on the parent's lap. Make a game of it all and satisfy any curiosity expressed by the child.

Circulation and cardiovascular system
- Normal heart rate ranges are 95–140 beats/min (>160 tachycardia).

- Normal systolic blood pressure ranges are 80–115 mmHg (depends on age). The fall in heart rate means that the first and second heart sounds can be more carefully assessed. Murmurs are common in this age group, most of which will be benign.

Abdomen

If the child is on a bed or couch it is important to make sure that a parent is near the head end. Kneel down and make sure the child's eye level is above yours and look at the child's face, not the belly.

Leg posture and gait are a frequent source of parental anxiety. Hip joint may be a focus of concern because of a limp or leg, thigh or knee pain. The limits of external and internal rotation can help decide what needs further evaluation.

Breathing and respiration

- Normal respiratory rate ranges are 20–30 breaths/min (>40 tachypnoea). Observe chest shape and respiratory pattern. Peak flow measurements are not reproducible until aged 4–5 years.

Neurology and development

Gait and gross motor abilities are assessed by play. Fine motor abilities can be assessed with a pencil and paper, by asking the child to copy various shapes: a circle by age 3 years, a cross by 4 years, a square by 4 years 6 months and triangles by 5 years. Hearing can be checked using games with free field audiometry. Social and behavioural skills are observed.

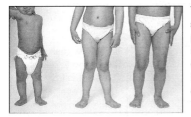

Three boys' legs. The youngest has slight genu varus (bow legs) which is physiological in the toddler. The middle brother has genu valgus (knock knees) which is physiological in the preschool-aged child. The eldest brother has 'straight' legs.

The actual neurological examination is somewhere between what was described for toddlers and a more adult format, so long as the child perceives your examination as a game.

THE SCHOOL CHILD

This is the age at which psychological factors can play a bigger role in how and what the child may complain of to their parents and doctor. Normal ranges for school-age children are:

- Heart rate – 80–120 beats/min (>140 tachycardia)

- Systolic blood pressure – 85–120 mmHg (depends on age)
- Respiratory rate – 15–20 breaths/min (>30 tachypnoea)

GROWTH

The height will usually be following near the midparental centile. Accelerations in height velocity may be due to an excessive weight gain or to endocrine causes. Decelerations may be due to unrecognised chronic illness or endocrine problems.

DEVELOPMENT

Children spend most of their day at school. Social and behavioural aspects are now most important. Language and cognitive skills, literacy and numeracy are further developed in class and at home. Vision, hearing and motor skills are approaching adult abilities.

HISTORY

Invite the child to be the historian. Pitch the questions in terms the child understands and which are not patronising.

Background information about home and especially school is important. How much does the presenting complaint affect the child's life at school? If only school time is affected then the problem may not be an organic one.

EXAMINATION

There are now very few differences in technique from examining adults, except that the examination should continue to be fun. Peak flow can be used as a reproducible way of monitoring asthma.

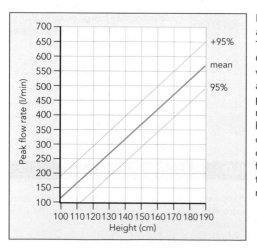

Peak flow chart according to height. These data from Godfrey et al. are valuable in predicting an expected range for peak expiratory flow rate according to height. Most 5 year olds can be taught to do reproducible peak flows, which can help in the diagnosis and monitoring of asthma.

ADOLESCENTS

Adolescent patients are a specific group and are distinct from all other groups, child or adult. There are many reasons for this:

- Adolescents seldom consult their doctor, so neither are very familiar with each other.
- Adolescents are uncertain as to how to behave as adults, but do not want to behave as children.
- Doctors need to accept that the adolescent is easily embarrassed and often anxious.
- The presenting problems can have a psychological basis.
- Adolescents with a chronic illness will demonstrate normal adolescent rebellion which can have serious long-term health consequences.
- Risk-taking behaviour (cigarettes, alcohol, drugs, sex and so on) is normal and it is hard not to appear judgmental and authoritative as their doctor.
- Deliberate self-harm (overdosages especially) is becoming more prevalent. Understanding the reasons for this behaviour can be challenging.
- Confidentiality and consent are sometimes a source of conflict between patient and parent and doctor.
- It is good practice to communicate effectively with both the adolescent and parents.

GROWTH

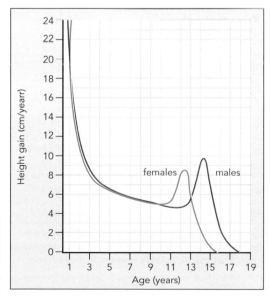

Height velocity in girls and boys. Note how before the pubertal growth spurt there is little difference in girls and boys height velocities. Also note that girls pubertal height velocity peaks are earlier and less tall than that for boys. These are thought to be the main factors determining the difference in adult male and female height.

PUBERTY

The onset of puberty is less than 1 year apart in girls and boys, but the pubertal growth spurt occurs in girls approxiamtely 2 years before boys. The first physical sign of puberty in a girl is the development of breast tissue under the nipples; the first physical sign in boys is the enlargement of the testes. A boy's growth spurt does not occur until the testicular volume is approximately 10 ml.

In girls, the height velocity decelerates to less than 4 cm per year then the menarche occurs. Final adult height is achieved when the bony epiphyses fuse in the vertebrae and along the long bones of the leg. It is impossible to evaluate an adolescent's growth without knowledge of what stage of pubertal development they have reached.

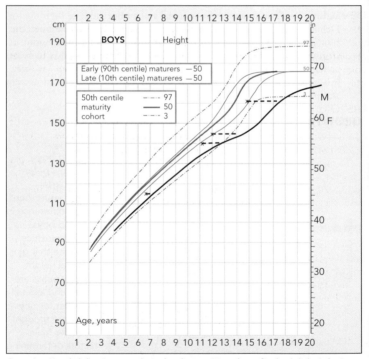

Constitutional delay in growth and puberty. Note how final adult height is near the tenth centile as predicted by the growth velocity observed between age 4 and 10 years. He was most psychologically stressed in his 16th year.

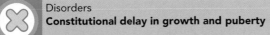

- This condition is most common in boys
- Patients usually have a history of growing in the lower quartile of the normal range but by the middle teenage years are very much shorter than their peers (at this time they present to a specialist clinic)
- Severe psychological stress may result from this genetic and physiological delay in puberty
- Augmenting puberty is an effective way of relieving the stress suffered by these patients

DEVELOPMENT

Development continues long after growth has finished. The gap between the end of growth and the end of development into a fully independent adult is apparently widening. The mean age for pubertal milestones appears to have come down from that of a century ago. The end of 'development' is often only complete after the age of 20 years.

HISTORY

This is one area in which confidentiality and consent may become a point of conflict. When taking the history, it is important to direct your questions primarily to the patient and only when necessary to the parent or carer.

Details about the family and relationships between members of the household are important. Details about school, progress with school work, hobbies, sports, pastimes and friendships can all help give an indication of how the adolescent is coping with the increasing stresses of the real world.

EXAMINATION

Most adolescents are very self-conscious of their appearance, so make sure they have suitable facilities to prevent undue embarrassment. The examining doctor will need to decide during the history taking whether the parent is to be invited alongside the patient. Which side of the screens should the parent stay? This can be difficult to get right every time.

Apart from the assessment of growth and puberty and attention to the adolescent and parent relationship, the examination will be similar to that for an adult patient.

Normal ranges for adolescents are:
- Heart rate – 60–100 beats/min (>120 tachycardia)
- Systolic blood pressure – 100–140 mmHg (depends on sex, size and age)
- Respiratory rate – 15–20 breaths/min (>30 tachypnoea)